Globalisation, Markets and Healthcare Policy

Although the last two decades have seen the healthcare systems of most developed countries face pressure for major reform, the impact of this reform on the relationship between empowerment, consumerism and citizen's rights has received limited research attention. *Globalisation, Markets and Healthcare Policy* sets out to redress this imbalance.

This book explores the extent to which globalisation and commercialisation relate to current and emerging health policies. It also looks at the implications for citizens, patients and social rights, as well as how policy making interacts with the interests of global and European trade and economic policies. Topics discussed include:

- How the impact of globalisation on health systems is apparent in the influence of international actors and European policies
- How the impact of globalisation is mediated by national priorities and policies
- How commercialisation of health is presented as benefiting citizens and patients but has the potential to undermine the aims and values inherent in health systems
- How the role of citizens' interests, social rights, patients' rights and priorities of patient and public involvement need to be separated from commercialisation, choice and consumerism in healthcare.

Essential reading for policy makers and students of public policy, politics, law and health services, *Globalisation, Markets and Healthcare Policy* will also appeal to those interested in patient involvement, international healthcare, international relations, transnational organisations and the EU.

Jonathan Tritter is Research Professor in Patient and Public Involvement, Special Advisor in the NHS Centre for Involvement at the University of Warwick and Professorial Fellow in the Governance and Public Management Group in Warwick Business School.

Meri Koivusalo is Senior Researcher in the National Institute for Health and Welfare (THL), Finland.

Eeva Ollila is Senior Researcher in the National Institute for Health and Welfare (THL), Finland and Adjunct Professor of Health Policy at the University of Tampere, Finland.

Paul Dorfman is Senior Research Fellow at the NHS Centre for Involvement at the University of Warwick.

Critical Studies in Health and Society
Series Editors
Simon J. Williams and Gillian Bendelow

This major new international book series takes a critical look at health in a rapidly changing social world. The series includes theoretically sophisticated and empirically informed contributions on cutting-edge issues from leading figures within the sociology of health and allied disciplines and domains. Other titles in the series include:

Contesting Psychiatry
Social movements in mental health
Nick Crossley

Lifestyle in Medicine
Gary Easthope and Emily Hansen

Medical Sociology and Old Age
Towards a sociology of health in later life
Paul Higgs and Ian Rees Jones

Emotional Labour in Health Care
The unmanaged heart of nursing
Catherine Theodosius

Globalisation, Markets and Healthcare Policy
Redrawing the patient as consumer
Jonathan Tritter, Meri Koivusalo, Eeva Ollila and Paul Dorfman

Written in a lively, accessible and engaging style, with many thought-provoking insights, the series will cater to a truly interdisciplinary audience of researchers, professionals, practitioners and policy makers with an interest in health and social change.

Those interested in submitting proposals for single or co-authored, edited or co-edited volumes should contact the series editors, Simon J. Williams (s.j.williams@warwick.ac.uk) and Gillian Bendelow (g.a.bendelow@ sussex.ac.uk).

Globalisation, Markets and Healthcare Policy

Redrawing the patient as consumer

Jonathan Tritter
Meri Koivusalo
Eeva Ollila
Paul Dorfman

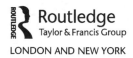
Routledge
Taylor & Francis Group

LONDON AND NEW YORK

First published 2010 by Routledge
2 Park Square, Milton Park, Abingdon, Oxon, OX14 4RN

Simultaneously published in the USA and Canada
by Routledge
270 Madison Ave, New York NY 10016

*Routledge is an imprint of the Taylor & Francis Group,
an informa business*

Transferred to Digital Printing 2010

Typeset in Sabon by Swales and Willis Ltd, Exeter, Devon

British Library Cataloguing in Publication Data
A catalogue record for this book is available
from the British Library

Library of Congress Cataloging in Publication Data
Tritter, Jonathan Q., 1965-
Globalisation, markets, and healthcare policy: redrawing
the patient as consumer / Jonathan Tritter, Meri Koivusalo, Eeva Ollila.
p.; cm. — (Critical studies in health and society)
Includes bibliographical references.
1. Medical policy. 2. Medical economics. 3. Globalization.
4. Right to health care. I. Koivusalo, Meri, 1964– II. Ollila, Eeva, 1959–
III. Title. IV. Series: Critical studies in health and society.
[DNLM: 1. Health Policy—economics—Europe. 2. Health Policy—trends—Europe.
3. Internationality—Europe. 4. Marketing of Health Services—economics—Europe.
5. Marketing of Health Services—trends—Europe. 6. Patient Participation—
economics—Europe. 7. Patient Participation—trends—Europe.
WA 525 T839g 2009]
RA394.T75 2009
338.4'73621—dc22
2008055418

ISBN10: 0–415–41702–3 (hbk)
ISBN10: 0–415–61205–5 (pbk)
ISBN10: 0–203–87509–5 (ebk)

ISBN13: 978–0–415–41702–0 (hbk)
ISBN13: 978–0–415–61205–0 (pbk)
ISBN13: 978–0–203–87509–4 (ebk)

Contents

Illustrations

Acknowledgements

We would like to acknowledge the Academy of Finland and the Ministry of Social Affairs and Health for funding the *Globalisation and Citizens in Health Care: Exploring the role of users, choice and markets in Europe* Project.

We would also like to acknowledge our host organisations, the Globalism and Social Policy Programme at the Finnish National Research and Development Centre for Welfare and Health (STAKES, since 2009 the National Institute for Health and Welfare), the Governance and Public Management Group at Warwick Business School and the NHS Centre for Involvement at the University of Warwick for supporting our work and enabling us to pursue a critical agenda.

We would like to recognise and thank Anna Alanko who supported the work of the project in numerous ways and Riitta-Maija Hämäläinen for her help in the latter stages of the project.

We would also like to acknowledge the contribution of members of the Project Advisory Board.

We would like to thank the many and diverse insiders who were good enough to speak with us, formally and informally, during the course of this study. Your openness and reflections on past, present and future have helped guide our thinking.

Acknowledgements

Introduction
The basis of the book

This book grew from the observation that across Europe the development of health policy appeared to be incorporating two distinct and sometimes mutually exclusive ideas: a process of healthcare reform promoting competition and the commercialisation of services on the one hand and a focus on citizen and patient rights and their involvement in the evaluation and development of health services on the other. Both discourses are drawn on to support *patient choice* as a further mechanism for health reform but they do so from entirely different justifications.

These two apparently distinct discourses suggest very different visions of a publicly funded health system. The first, promoting a system built on competition between service providers and separation of funding from provision of health services. In such a system opportunities are created for a range of different public, private and voluntary sector actors. The benefits claimed for this model are that competition brings cost-containment and increased quality in provision. The second discourse marries patient-centred care and the role and rights of the individual patient in decisions about their own care with local, regional and national opportunities for citizens to help shape the organisation and delivery of publicly funded health services.

During the last two decades the healthcare systems of most developed countries have faced pressure for major reform. The perceived problems facing healthcare systems – increasing costs, inefficiency, inflexibility, poor management – as well as the nature of the suggested reforms – management reforms, cost-containment measures, contracting out – have, across different national contexts, exhibited many similarities in design (OECD 1992; 1994; 1996; Drache and Sullivan 1999). The *first wave of healthcare reforms* was implemented in the 1980s and early 1990s. These were inspired and guided, to a large extent, by the concept of 'internal markets' in healthcare and drew on the insights of Enthoven as well as the work of the Organisation for Economic Co-operation and Development (OECD) on public sector management and healthcare reforms (Enthoven 1989; Ham and Brommels 1994; Moran and Wood 1996).

We observed that in countries as distinct as the Netherlands, England, Sweden and Finland these discourses had a high profile and were the touchstones and justification for radical reform of the publicly funded health system (Harrison 2004). We wondered if we were seeing evidence of a *second wave of healthcare reforms* in which a discourse emphasising economic efficiency and cost-containment was losing dominance to other agendas (Koivusalo and Tritter 2006) such as patient-centred care and consumerism.

In this book we also focus on the nature and ways in which a *second wave of healthcare reform* incorporating a more private-sector oriented phase inspired by other policy areas including trade, competition and industry appears to be taking place. The issue is no longer about internal markets or making public services more effective, but seeking to incorporate competition and ensuring a 'level playing field' for private sector providers. We were interested in how this new wave of reforms is linked to and reinforces additional pressure for increased competition and commercialisation in healthcare services and prompts patient consumerism as a central driving mechanism. And further what the role different global and regional agendas, actors and processes play in the changes observed in each country. We consider to what extent choice and the promotion of mechanisms of choice are a crucial part of a *second wave of healthcare reforms* and the influence of the emphasis on internal markets and the four freedoms of the European Union. Has the context of health policy changed and can we explain similarities and differences in policies?

We were interested in identifying how policy ideas, rhetoric and discourse travelled between countries. That is, we saw the emergence of common justifications for health policy reform in different countries as not simply a product of policy transfer but perhaps an example of globalisation. Further, if this was an example of globalisation were some actors more effective mediators for policy messages than others?

This book reflects a genuinely European focus as the European Union agenda on health has been developing quickly and a focus solely on individual countries would not allow us to engage with the broader set of challenges that European legal policy developments pose for health systems. We consider the European Union both as a mediator of global and 'globalisation' pressures as well as a distinct forum on its own terms. Health reform processes, particularly in European countries, can be understood in the context of continued European Community integration and global trade negotiations that are increasingly focused on broad economic, legislative and regulatory issues and extend their influence and remit over healthcare services (Koivusalo 2003a; 2003b). However, it is also about the development of the European Union as a global actor in the context of the Lisbon Strategy, *European Governance* (Commission of the European Union 2001) and an emphasis on 'European citizens', as reflected in the continued debate over the reform and development of the next EU Treaty.

While globalisation might well play a role in promoting and transmitting policy ideas and solutions, it is the political mechanisms within individual nation states that have an even bigger role in defining policy content and shaping implementation. One important aspect of our study was the way in which different actors within states understood and responded to the discourses on commercialisation of health services and the promotion of patient involvement. We were interested, in particular, in the role of civil servants in the health ministry, health professionals' associations (unions), health voluntary organisations and key opinion formers (government advisors, academics and think tanks) and the ways in which they would relate their advice emerging from the global and European context on domestic policy issues.

This set the stage for a study of three countries within Europe that shared some common characteristics in the nature and shape of their publicly funded health system. Finland, Sweden and England all maintain national health services that are premised on universal access, primarily public provision, and funded mainly through national taxation. In all three countries state provision is the dominant form of health delivery but there are some private sector actors and all three states have adopted some form of co-payment. There was much that was different between the three countries – population size and diversity, orientation towards the European Union, structure and accountability for health service provision.

The purpose of our study was not to explore variations in health systems in Europe, but to focus on the ways in which health policy and reforms relating to marketisation and user involvement had evolved in these three states. However, in contrast to more traditional focus on historical institutionalism emphasizing on the institutional contexts for policies and policy change, we have adopted a deliberately global policy focus with an emphasis on commonalities. We explore the extent to which globalisation, European or global influences can be seen as explanatory factors in the process of health policy reform and the extent to which this is recognised by national policy actors.

Our approach in each country was to review the literature and documentation on health policy between 1985 and 2005. We did both documentary and literature search in the areas and covered documents in three languages (English, Swedish and Finnish). This helped us to identify key stakeholders within the different categories of influence (policy makers, civil servants, health professional associations, voluntary organisations and academic critics/advisors). Interviewing these key stakeholders helped us understand the process, evolution, intent and impact of health policy discourses relating to commercialisation and involvement. Overall we interviewed more than 50 stakeholders across the three countries, the European Union and international organisations.

In the next section we turn to consider some of the key terms that relate to the evolution of health policies we engage with before we move on to outline the contents and main arguments of the volume.

Health policy, healthcare reforms and health systems

This book focuses on the contents and process of setting a health policy agenda, rather than the implementation of policy and service delivery, in practice. In other words, our main interest is on why the particular ideas underpinning particular healthcare reforms became important, how these relate to the commercialisation of healthcare and how this relates to user involvement, choice and the promotion of citizens, consumers or patient rights. We recognise that the implementation of policy has a profound effect not only on those who use public services but also in shaping the views of voters and policy makers, creating a feedback loop that informs future policy. We also recognise that different policy fields interact and indeed decisions that impact on the healthcare arena are often not enacted directly within the health policy sector. However, the requirements for a meaningful analysis of policy implementation and practice are different and these could form the basis of further study in the future.

The concepts and understanding of terms such as health policy, healthcare reforms and health systems requires further elaboration. The second chapter in the book provides the basis for conceptual definition and articulation of health policy, healthcare reforms and health systems as well as covering some key aspects of similarities and difference in the three countries.

Globalisation and influence by global actors

Globalisation is a term used widely and with very different meanings (Scholte 2001; Held *et al.* 1999). In this book we choose to use the term globalisation to generally refer to economic globalisation in terms of a process of economic integration and the ways that different actors, legislative frameworks and forums have become empowered or disempowered in national policy debates. However, we also use globalisation in the context of the transnational transmission and mediation of ideas and processes and their spread, for example, through epistemic communities, and as a reference to policy diffusion and policy influence by global and regional agencies. This use of the term helps us to understand globalisation better in the context of policy development and as part of the broader policy process.

We focus in our analysis on the main ways in which globalisation, and in particular economic globalisation – economic integration – influences decisions made outside the traditional remit of health policy as well as health policy priorities and health practice. While we recognise the broader global aspects and importance of global change, migration, climate change and technological development that are often analysed as part of the impacts of globalisation, we seek a narrower remit.

We also choose not to focus as much on the implications or impacts of intellectual property rights on health policies and in particular pharmaceutical policies. We do want to underline that we think that further attention to this matter is required on the basis of studies of the application of public resources to pharmaceutical research and development. In this book, however, we have not explored these issues but instead directed our attention to the ways in which health policies are shaped. In other words, we focus on key aspects of change in particular for health services, which would have relevance to policy making and relate to the ways in which health policy and broader decisions within health systems are made.

As part of globalisation and the diffusion of ideas we explore how certain types of policy ideas have migrated between different stakeholders and shaped health policy in Finland, Sweden and England. The context and to some extent the results of these policies have differed between countries. However, our main interest is focused on the ways in which each of the countries has responded, rather than on seeking evidence of the convergence of social policy models or the magnitude of public spending on health as both of these factors are blind to commercialisation processes.

Commercialisation of health services

The term commercialisation in the context of this book is used both to describe the engagement of commercial providers in the provision of publicly funded services as well as the regulatory framework and priorities which shape provision of services by both public and private providers. Our focus is thus broader than the traditional understanding of privatisation in terms of not concentrating merely on the private financing of healthcare. We also attend to the extent to which commercialisation takes place *within publicly provided and/or financed services* as consequence of reform policies on the basis of an increased role for the private sector in provision. Further we explore how aims, priorities and regulatory measures are set within health policy. In this context we have tried to narrow our focus to the drivers of policy change and the ways in which aspects of patient choice or patient, citizen and user involvement have been part of this process.

Consumerism in health services

We define consumerism in health services as the means and mechanisms that enhance processes and practices that rely on active choices made by individual service users. In health services we can also see examples of indirect consumerism, where agents for individual service users are given more power to act in healthcare markets. We also explore how consumerist incentives towards creating more demanding patients as part of their care operate in the context of the advertising of services, medicines and treatments. Similarly, how such tendencies create a requirement for healthcare organisations and healthcare systems to respond to patient demands and needs in relation to treatments for which there is a limited, lacking or contrasting evidence-base is also explored. In other words we explore the extent to which consumerism redefines the basis of healthcare services not in terms of needs, impact and clinical value of treatments, but in terms of consumer demands.

Health service consumerism is often associated with the commercialisation of health services, but it is important to note that privatisation or commercialisation of services can take place in a context with only limited or indirect consumerism. Furthermore we can also see health service consumerism as part of a broader process of selling services to healthy people, such as LASIK surgery, cosmetic dentistry or other aspects of cosmetic surgery. However, this more commercialised context of service provision is not our core interest as our focus is on services in general.

The 'choice agenda' in the public sector is crucial to the promotion of markets in service provision and the redefinition of the 'service user' as consumer. Recent examples of choice policies have related to schools and are increasingly being applied to publicly funded healthcare. Swedish legislation under the central conservative government has sought to promote opportunities for greater individual patient choice. Opportunities for consumerism are predicated on sufficient surplus in the health system to allow for selection; patient choice is dependent on economic inefficiency. The risk-pooling upon which public provision of health services depends is undermined by individual choice as it limits the subsidisation of the long-term and seriously ill by the young and well. Finally, in terms of prioritisation, the provision of services that an individual would seek for themselves is likely to be very different from those services that an individual feels are most appropriate for their community or collective benefit.

We seek to distinguish between consumer interest in health services and consumerism; the latter is based on the assumptions and priority of a sovereign consumer in a market place while consumer interests do not necessarily imply consumerism in healthcare. In contrast, at the population level some consumer interests can best be served by a less consumerism-driven healthcare context. The consumer interests in healthcare relate to quality, safety and price of services and possibilities for complaints, redress and compensation when problems are faced.

Patient and public involvement

Sometimes referred to as user involvement this issue seeks to create a different relationship between those who receive or could receive health services and those who plan and provide those services. Covering a range of different relationships, involvement activities aim to ensure that decisions about the planning, organisation and delivery of services take in to account the views, experiences and wishes of those for whom the services are intended. Further, that the process of decision making about the prioritisation and availability of services includes members of the public. There are other categories of involvement from the training of healthcare professionals, setting research agendas, and decisions about individual care and treatment plans but the same principle of 'nothing about us without us' applies.

For some scholars patient and public involvement is a mechanism to promote civil society renewal and greater democratic accountability while for others it is about the shifting of responsibility from professionals to lay people; from self-selected elite to an unrepresentative, unelected minority of the public. While patient involvement often deals with patient–doctor interaction our focus in this book is on a broader level about the policy and planning context. We discuss both hard and soft mechanisms to promote patient and public involvement and the context in which these take place.

Citizens' rights and public involvement

Our book is not a legal analysis of health services related to human, social or patient rights nor does it intend to cover broader discourses on deliberative democracy or participation. However, we have found it important to include some aspects of these issues as it is important to understand the ways in which policies on patient and public involvement are set out and emerge as part of a broader framework of national, regional and global commitments. Human and social rights stipulations, for example, have been conducive to the consideration of patient rights and public involvement. Patient rights are also different from citizen's rights to access healthcare, something which is not always apparent in practice.

Public involvement in this context is a form of accountability, but also relates to how power is shared and enacted. A policy shift towards embracing public participation and a stakeholder society can also take place in a context where democratic accountability is weakened. A further aspect of stakeholder participation is that it tends to include particular corporate-sector interest organisations and lobbying groups that are also defined as stakeholders resulting in a very diverse conceptualisation in practice of a citizen focus. On the other hand, the emphasis on patient and public participation may also take place independently of democratic accountability or governance. One example of conflicting interests and governance has been the enhanced role of industry funded patient organisations (such as Consumer Powerhouse) in European policy making and the ways in which this may undermine the democratic accountability of national and local governments.

The structure of the book

This book explores how the tensions between commercialisation, consumerism and patient and public involvement in healthcare have emerged in health policy debates over the last 20 years. We illustrate the different views and interests of categories of stakeholders in three countries – England, Finland and Sweden – as well as within the broader context of the European Union. We also seek to understand the role of international organisations such as the OECD and World Health Organisation (WHO) in shaping, transmitting and promoting certain kinds of policy ideas. The overall argument of the book explores the extent to which globalisation and commercialisation relate to current and emerging health policies and the implications for citizens, patients and social rights. Further, how policy making interacts with the interests of global trade and economic policies to shape an increasingly mobile professional workforce and an international market for patients and healthcare providers is also explored.

The book is divided into three sections: the evolution of key issues in health policies; case studies of England, Finland and Sweden; broader lessons and implications for policy making and critical analysis. In the first section Jonathan Tritter explores the development of patient and public involvement in healthcare (Chapter 1), with Paul Dorfman moving on to consider the shift from collective involvement to consumerism and patient choice (Chapter 3). In Chapter 2 Meri Koivusalo outlines the key components of a national health system and the organisation, institutional setting and financing of health services, and then goes on to highlight particular forms of commercialisation. With Eeva Ollila, she then turns in Chapter 4 to the linkages between global and regional actors on health policy, commercial policy and health systems at a national level, and the implications of the changing political and financial context on the organisational structures and financial framework of health systems. The final chapter in the first section (Chapter 5) provides an opportunity for Meri Koivusalo to discuss the ways in which the European Union and, in particular, the evolving nature of internal market regulation and competence of European Commission influence national health policy priorities and practice.

The second section of the book builds on the first through the use of more detailed empirical evidence and insights from case studies of three countries, England (Chapter 6), Finland (Chapter 7) and Sweden (Chapter 8). The case studies have been collected as part of a larger study of *Globalisation and citizens in healthcare: Exploring the role of users, choice and markets in European health systems,* funded by the Academy of Finland and the Finnish Ministry of Health and Social Affairs. Jonathan Tritter and Paul Dorfman conducted the English case study, Meri Koivusalo and Eeva Ollila the Finnish case study while Meri Koivusalo and Jonathan Tritter are responsible for the Swedish case study. The focus on the three countries enables us in Chapter 9 to explore the commonalities and differences in the role and intent of stakeholders in influencing policy change in these three national contexts and what this reveals about broader globalising forces that shape the direction of health policy.

In the final chapter (Chapter 10) we conclude by raising critical issues in relation to future of health systems in these countries and implications of markets for equity and sustainability of national healthcare systems and how interests between the rights of citizens, patients and consumers differ. We also return to a discussion of globalisation and the need for an improved articulation of the common challenges to health systems. This chapter provides an overall analysis and a focus on the evolution of policies and policy articulation and the articulation of how globalisation relates to given processes.

1 Analysing patient and public involvement and health policy

Recent health service reforms in Western countries emphasise public and patient involvement (Vallgårda *et al.* 2001; Vos 2002). The increasing participation of users in decisions around treatment, service development and evaluation has been central to this process. The consequences are becoming clear as relationships between the state and citizens and between the public, patients and organisations within the healthcare system are redrawn. This shift in health policy has generated significant debate between policy makers, within government and the media.

What is patient and public involvement?

Patient and Public Involvement (PPI) is about creating a constructive dialogue to reshape the relationship between patients, healthcare professionals and the public. It has the potential to act as a catalyst for more widespread cultural change. Involvement activities should create an environment that enables issues to be raised by patients and the public and to be fed into strategic and operational decisions in order to change policy and practice, and at an individual level ensure that patient views and experiences have an impact on decision making regarding treatment, the training of health professionals and the generation of research evidence. According to the UK Department of Health (2008a) members of the public should have a substantial role in shaping the care system's development, and patients and service users should be kept well informed of clinical processes and decisions.

Building successful relationships between those that use or receive services, those who commission or plan services and those who manage or deliver services is essential to ensure efficient and effective service provision that meets the needs of service users. In healthcare the promotion of patient-centred or holistic care seeks to ensure that a patient's needs and views are central to decisions about treatment and care. In a publicly funded health system the need to ensure accountability to those who fund services (the taxpaying public) and the political necessity of satisfying voters informs the opportunities that exist for patient and public involvement. These different ways of framing various accountability relationships assume that the quality of health services is inexorably linked to meeting the expressed needs of both patients and the public; responding to the views of both individual service users and the collective population.

Theories of user empowerment are often traced to Arnstein's (1969) classic article setting out a 'ladder of citizen engagement'. Her work has been applied and reinterpreted in a number of ways and indeed recent criticisms have focused on the polarisation between the interest of citizens (service users) and public sector managers inherent in her model (Tritter and McCallum 2006) rather than exploring the opportunities for partnership and the identification and promotion of a common agenda (Moore 1995).

An urban redevelopment specialist, Arnstein developed and illustrated her typology of citizen participation in decision making with examples from the US Department of Housing and Urban Development Modern Cities programme. She suggested, however, that her model was more broadly relevant: 'The underlying issues are essentially the same – "nobodies" in several arenas are trying to become "somebodies" with enough power to make the target institutions responsive to their views, aspirations, and needs' (Arnstein 1969: 216).

Arnstein suggests a 'Ladder of citizen participation' but the primary measure of participation is power to make decisions and seizing this control is the true aim of citizen engagement and the extent of such power differentiates between the different rungs of the ladder. Thus, complete citizen control is defined as the top of the ladder. Moving from the lower rungs labelled *manipulation* and *therapy* through *informing*, *consultation* and *placation* to the top three steps, *partnership*, *delegated power* and *citizen control*, demonstrates citizen power. Lower rungs are differentiated by the constraint of citizen power and forms of participation that does not necessarily influence decision making.

In healthcare the two categories of patients and the public tend to be defined only vaguely. The public is often seen to represent or serve as a proxy for potential patients while at other times it is seen as synonymous with citizens, taxpayers and voters. In a UK Department of Health Report, public involvement is defined as 'the participation of members of the public or their representatives, in decisions about the planning, design and development of their local health services' (Farrell 2004: 66). For Coulter the differentiation between patients and the public is more significant: 'All of us are both patients, or potential patients, and citizens, but a distinction can usefully be made between what we want when we are using the health service and what we hope for as citizens or taxpayers' (Coulter 2006: 38). This distinction is partly around the tension between engaging with individual patients and engaging with people as part of a collective, citizens, to whom public services are accountable. Reflecting on this tension within the UK Coulter goes on to observe

> Involving citizens means opening up debate about the pattern and nature of service provision, while engaging patients involves tackling the clinical

agenda and changing the culture of care . . . . while considerable efforts have been expended on consulting local people about planned service developments and securing lay membership on a raft of committees and policy-making bodies, progress in respect of involving patients in their care has been disappointingly slow.

(Coulter 2006: 39)

The category of patients typically also includes a range of other collective terms reflecting those who are directly affected by health services, including carers, service users, consumers of services and lay people. UK Department of Health defines patient involvement as 'the full participation of patients and their carers in their own care and treatment. Patient involvement can also be at the level of service delivery and quality monitoring' (Farrell 2004: 66).

A further complicating issue relates to time. How long does an individual retain the definition of patient? An individual who receives a prescription for a two-week course of antibiotics for a chest infection is no longer a *patient* in the sense of being actively treated a month later. A patient who has a hip replacement will expect to drive within four to six weeks and feel normal after about three months. A patient who has a lumpectomy for breast cancer should be able to resume regular activities six weeks after surgery. A patient who is diagnosed with asthma will typically manage their condition with inhalers. Of these examples how many would still be considered 'patients' two years after the completion of their treatment?

The person with cancer may continue to think of themselves as a *cancer patient* or living with cancer long after an initial diagnosis and treatment, even if their contact with health professionals is limited to an annual check-up. Similarly, a person with a hip replacement continues to be aware of the surgical intervention. Some people with long-term or chronic conditions reject the label of patient despite maintaining an ongoing relationship with healthcare professionals to aid the management of their condition.

The overlapping categories of patient and the public also incorporate a second order definition that relates to the intensity and regularity of contact with a health system. Further, being a *cancer patient* provides a particular expertise about cancer services but does not imply any broader general knowledge of local health services. The relationships between people, the health system and those who provide healthcare reflect the different types of potential partnerships and therefore different kinds of involvement.

Different categories of patient and public involvement

In the UK, the Department of Health's Patient Partnership Strategy laid out a series of different kinds of 'partnerships' with distinct aims to:

[P]romote patients' involvement in their own health and healthcare as active partners with professionals; enable patients to have information about their health and healthcare and to make informed decisions about it if they wish; involve users and their carers in improving service quality; and involve the public as citizens in health and health service decision making processes.

(Department of Health 1999a: 2)

These different partnerships reflect to an extent the distinction between patients and the public as well as the type of involvement. More explicitly, there are five distinct types of patient and public involvement (see Table 1.1).

Patient participation in treatment decisions is one type of user involvement but as a form of patient-centred care it is not innovative. Similarly, involvement in service development, typically a consultation exercise with a local community, has a long history in the NHS and more broadly around the world. The evaluation of services by users has become common practice. Information, in England can be obtained from, for instance, the Patient Advice and Liaison Service (PALS) and from Non-Executive Directors (and Citizen Governors in Foundation Trusts) that are all important avenues for ensuring that the views of the public and patients can inform strategic and operational decision making. Two final categories of user involvement relate to participation in research and teaching.

Clearly, there are interactions and linkages between the different categories of user involvement. Service development may have a direct impact on the range of individual treatment options that exist and service evaluation may identify inequities in access that affect individual participation in treatment. User participation in setting a research agenda may have an impact on shaping provision and service organisation, and therefore future options for treatment (Involve 2003).

A second key distinction to draw between types of PPI is whether they are direct or indirect (Tritter *et al.* 2003). *Direct involvement* occurs when people take part directly in decision making. This includes determining what

Table 1.1 Types of patient and public involvement

Type of involvement	Patient	Public	Example
Involvement in decisions about treatment and care	✓		Prostatectomy or radiotherapy
Involvement in service development	✓	✓	Prioritising or commissioning/purchasing services
Involvement in the evaluation of service provision	✓		Patient satisfaction survey
Involvement in teaching/training health professionals	✓		Social impact of diabetes
Involvement in health research	✓	✓	Identifying relevant research questions

services are offered to a particular population, improvements needed to the quality of services, and how resources are used in relation to prioritisation.

There are a variety of methods for involving people directly in decision making; for example, by having patients or members of the public on steering groups and committees at different levels within an organisation. Alternatively, organising 'User Involvement Groups' to help advise on policy development and decision making within a healthcare organisation is a common approach. These groups typically have members drawn from professional groups, support groups and service users and they can provide a useful forum for bringing together different experiences, perspectives and expertise.

By contrast, *indirect involvement* often entails information gathering by health professionals and clinical staff in order to inform service delivery and development. While the views of people are sought, health professionals and clinical staff make the final decisions. One of the difficulties with indirect engagement is that health professionals and managerial staff can choose to ignore feedback from people if they do not think it is appropriate. As a result, those who have contributed to the process can feel frustrated. However, by providing clear feedback about how and why decisions have been taken, these feelings may be reduced. The vast majority of involvement in healthcare is indirect involvement where the power to make a decision is reserved for those with formal responsibility; an approach that is far lower on Arnstein's ladder (Arnstein 1969).

As well as the five types of user involvement suggested earlier in the chapter (treatment decisions, service development, evaluation of services, education and training or research) and the distinction between direct and indirect approaches, a further distinction can be drawn between those activities that are aimed at individuals and those that are premised on collective participation (see Figure 1.1). For individuals, an example of direct involvement might be choosing to have a particular procedure, or choosing not to have chemotherapy. Collective direct involvement might be involving a breast cancer support group in designing a new breast cancer clinic in a local hospital. In each of these cases the involvement activity includes the power to participate in making the decision.

Individual Direct	Individual Indirect
Collective Direct	Collective Direct

Figure 1.1 A matrix of involvement

Examples of indirect involvement at the individual level include making a complaint or providing input about a positive experience of care. At a collective level indirect involvement might be the comments by a patient support group about their recommendations for service improvement in reaction to a draft report. In all these cases the involvement activity generates information, but the decision to act on the information, and indeed what aspects of the information to take into account, is retained by the health professional or manager.

Proactive and reactive involvement

A final element of this conceptual model of involvement relates to the extent to which involvement activities are prompted. Many health organisations have recognised that developing and supporting service user groups is beneficial in generating relevant intelligence on service design, and helping to target resources and services to the needs of the local community. Such groups, whether they are health or citizen panels (Somerset Health and Social Care NHS Trust 2008; Davies *et al.* 2006), or an involvement forum (London Ambulance Service 2004), will operate in different ways. The health organisation is likely to seek service user's views on plans or documents and send them to the group for review and feedback. Other organisations may ensure that the service user group has representatives on the board of the organisation and that there is a standing agenda item at every meeting that creates an opportunity for the group to raise issues that require a response (Avon, Somerset and Wiltshire Cancer Services 2006).

Whatever methods are used and whichever type of PPI is employed, it must relate to both the aims of the activity or system of involvement and the type of people involved.

Are complaints jewels to be treasured?

Sometimes complaints are seen as an involvement mechanism and a type of patient and public involvement. Usually complaints are collected at a central point, analysed and coordinated. Complaints can identify particular aspects of a service, including individuals, that are underperforming or that need to be addressed. Complaints, however, are unrepresentative of dissatisfaction and do not necessarily capture the most serious grievances or instances of inappropriate practice (Mulcahy and Tritter 1998). This makes them a poor tool to monitor services.

While complaints may be a form of user activism (Mulcahy and Lloyd-Bostock 1994) they can only form part of indirect involvement as they are framed in terms of *collecting information* rather than participation in decision making. The action taken in response to a complaint, usually, is made without the participation of the complainant. Complaints also tend to emphasise an individual relationship and tend to be single instances. They are therefore only limited opportunities for developing a partnership with a community

Lay expertise

All of these categories of user acknowledge specific expertise distinct from that available to health professionals and managers. While this has been stressed most strongly in relation to chronic illness and the promotion of self-management it also underpins the increasing stress of patient participation in treatment decision making and has been labelled by others as the 'autonomous patient' (Coulter 2002) or the 'resourceful patient' (Muir Gray and Rutter 2002).

Despite this there is much contestation of the nature and extent of such expertise (see, for instance, Shaw and Baker 2004). In launching the Expert Patient programme the Chief Medical Officer of England Professor Sir Liam Donaldson said,

> It has long been recognised that people with chronic diseases have considerable knowledge and experience of their own illness. Research has shown that with proper training this can be turned into practical skills to enable the patient to play a bigger part in managing their own condition . . . . The new Expert Patients Programme will help to create a new generation of patients who are empowered to take action with the health professional caring for them to, reduce pain, improve the use of medication and improve their overall quality of life. Patients will receive the support to help them take more control of their own health and treatment, to make more appropriate use of health and social services and feel empowered in their relationship with healthcare professionals.
>
> (Donaldson 2001)

This suggests that it is only when users are appropriately trained and supported that they can be regarded as 'experts'. More importantly patients and the public are experts by experience. Patients and carers have direct experience of the delivery of services and are ideally placed to identify problems and proffer solutions to the way they are organised and delivered.

Why involve patients and the public?

When involvement is done well a partnership develops between those responsible for delivering healthcare, those receiving it and those who fund it. At an individual patient level, involvement helps ensure patient-centred care and fully informed consent. As the proportion of healthcare related to long-term conditions increases the relevance of patient's experience also increases. Involving people in decisions about their own care on the basis of their own expertise about their long-term condition is essential and yields greater scope for co-production of wellbeing and increased likelihood that agreed treatment regimes will be followed (Bodenheimer *et al*. 2002). This key aspect has been championed by the promotion of patient rights (Active Citizenship Network 2002; International Alliance of Patient Organisations 2006) and framed by various sets of 'principles' of patient and public involvement (NHS Quality Improvement Scotland 2003; Lloyd and Cummins 2003; Health Canada 2000).

Decisions about the allocation of resources and the organisation and delivery of health services based on involvement are more legitimate. Those decisions will be made in the context of the priorities and experiences of patients and the relevant communities. The legitimacy of proposed changes generated through appropriate involvement limits resistance and lessens conflict (Arnstein 1969; Balducci and Fareri 1998; Appelstrand 2002).

Importantly, any of the plans and proposed changes will be made with the expertise of those with experience of both delivering and receiving services. Patient and public involvement helps ensure that different questions are asked and multiple perspectives are brought to bear on a particular decision; far broader discussions are enabled by the diversity of perspectives. Involvement also tends to focus on the experience and management of the process as well as outcomes. Helping to engineer a process that maximises satisfaction is likely to yield broader benefits.

Patient and public involvement is a key ingredient in the development and delivery of efficient and effective health services. Working with patients helps ensure that their experience – the lived patient pathway – is at the heart of how services are planned, organised and delivered. The outcomes of strategic decisions will be more acceptable to patients and the public if they have been involved and are likely to yield greater satisfaction and less resistance. For staff too, the knowledge that the way they are organising and delivering services is built on experience and shaped by patient and public preferences generates greater satisfaction.

Engagement for improvement

To improve and change healthcare services, healthcare organisations need to have robust engagement and consultation practices that:

- enable ongoing dialogue with local people,
- involve healthcare professionals and staff at every stage of the process, and
- are embedded into organisational decision-making processes.

These are key aspects of a systemic approach to patient and public involvement. Such an approach ensures that changes to healthcare services do not come as a surprise but are part of the life cycle of a health economy and that issues associated with unsafe care that emerge from the experience of patients can inform service improvement. Transparent and inclusive approaches to service design and redesign will ensure that the delivery of services adapts and responds to the changing needs and preferences of local people. Ongoing engagement and consultation is the foundation for shaping and facilitating improvements to healthcare services.

Not all reconfigurations are contentious and the degree of contentiousness is not always related to the scale of the change. It is heavily dependent on how well people understand why changes may have to be made and how much influence they have on the decisions that are taken. Evidence from many sources, including the public consultation on *Your Health, Your Care, Your Say* (Opinion Leader Research 2006), suggests that people will support difficult decisions when they are fully involved in the discussions and understand the reasons behind them.

The Chief Medical Officer of England, Professor Sir Liam Donaldson, in a recent address (Donaldson 2008) identified five different ways in which patient experience can act to improve health services. He argued that patients' experiences serve as the *conscience* of a system and *catalyst* for change. Patients are *witnesses* to the delivery of health services and can help shape the direction, like *compasses*, for change and improvement. Finally, patients can be *teachers* as their experiences are the consequences of the way services are delivered and often provide ways of doing things differently and better.

Patient and public involvement holds the promise of re-engineering a health system through systematic processes that ensure accountability and build partnerships between those who plan, manage and deliver health services and those who fund and receive them. Recognising this aim the UK Department of Health states:

> Real patient and public involvement is not about ticking boxes, it is about NHS organisations developing constructive relationships, building strong partnerships and communicating effectively. For patients' experiences of health services to really improve, NHS staff will need to have ongoing and meaningful dialogue with them, their carers and the public about improving and developing services .... [this] will strengthen accountability to patients and the public and make sure there is transparency and openness in decision-making procedures. We must develop and adapt health services around the needs of patients and the public which will build trust and confidence between local communities and the NHS.
>
> (Department of Health 2003b: 2)

An essential part of this re-engineering process is consciousness of what is occurring; a consciousness that is rarely separate from direct experience of involvement activities (Daykin *et al.* 2002). Those who have been 'involved', whether as patients or health professionals, typically approach their work in a different way in the future. It is this aspect of the process of patient and public involvement that endows it with the potential to change the culture of a health organisation. Building partnerships that share decision making at an individual doctor–patient level, engaging local communities in prioritising and planning health services and involving patients in drawing on their experience to improve services provide key ingredients for a systematic and continual process of multi-level accountability and improvement.

At the heart of the acknowledgement of the utility of involving users is the applicability of their particular experience and a perspective that is distinct from that of health professionals. But this experience too is subject to critique. The most typical response to the engagement with users is that they are not 'representative' of all users. This is often mirrored in the response that vocal health professionals are also not typical of their category. As Prior notes: 'Yet, experience on its own is rarely sufficient to understand the technical complexities of disease causation, its consequences or its management. This is partly because experiential knowledge is invariably limited, and idiosyncratic . . . Above all, lay people can be wrong' (2003: 53).

While acknowledging these limitations, the key contribution gained from involving patients and the public is founded in their distinct personal experience and non-medical or technical frame of reference; it is asking questions that health professionals have not considered. This suggests not a hierarchy of knowledge – relevant professional vs irrelevant lay – but rather a complementarity between forms of knowledge set within a willingness to acknowledge difference.

Theoretical justifications for patient and public involvement

The justification for patient and public involvement is predicated on a number of different theoretical bases but centrally the need for health services to be accountable to users as taxpayers, voters and consumers. These three aspects of accountability are highlighted in policy documents and are often used interchangeably.

Citizenship – the public as voters

Patient and public involvement grounded in local democratic processes, including local referenda, has been one of the more recent attempts to span the democratic deficit in the governance of publicly funded health services. In the UK this has been stressed most recently in the legislation on Foundation Trusts. The mandated approach seeks to ensure that current users' views about services are not prioritised over the views of local residents or those who work locally, who may be future users. Unfortunately, however, delegating power by expanding opportunities for electing local residents to be 'governors' of the hospital does not guarantee local accountability or engagement with the full spectrum of users. Local democratic processes and the *new localism* have several weaknesses that limit their ability to deliver user involvement (Pratchett 2004).

The *new localism* is associated with the UK New Labour government and is presented as a mechanism for delegating some power to communities; an attempt at decentralisation of decision making. It is championed in England by the New Local Government Network, a left-wing think tank with close ties to the British Labour Party founded in 1996 that 'seeks to transform public services, revitalise local political leadership and empower local communities' (New Local Government Network 2009). The impact of the agenda is apparent in pressure toward the personalisation of services and establishing mechanisms to support feedback from local communities to influence the nature, organisation and delivery of services. However, there is no strict definition of the *new localism* and as one commentator put it,

> No one is terribly precise about the nature of the beast, whether it means simply giving councils more power or money, reinventing local government or – fashionable this year in New Labour circles – pushing things down to the level of neighbourhoods or communities (another two words rarely defined).
>
> (Walker 2005)

Mechanisms to encourage local responsiveness do not necessarily rely on voting but are intended to provide a different model of accountability and variation in service provision based on expressed need.

Relying on local democratic processes may close off other options for user involvement because the voting is often seen as the highest form of user involvement despite evidence of low electoral turnout (Topf 1995; Fieldhouse, Tranmer and Russell 2007). As noted earlier, countries such as Finland and Sweden offer only limited opportunities for direct user involvement in health service policy and planning. Instead, elected members from local municipal governments appoint members of municipality and health service boards. Effective representation, however, requires a clear mandate, informed decisions by local people on key health issues and an ongoing process of active engagement with users and the public to ensure proper channels of communication. Without such assurances turnout rates for local elections are declining in many communities (Franklin 2004) and mobilisation appears to occur only in response to specific issues, for example, to protest against hospital closure.

In addition, expecting people to participate in formal election processes may exclude members of vulnerable populations that are both more likely to require health services and historically have been less well served. Such approaches may perpetuate institutional discrimination and existing power imbalances – for example, age, gender, income – by emphasising the election process over the need to include a representative range of views. This approach may be problematic in a culturally diverse society where not everyone shares a common understanding of dialectic-based approaches. Populations with limited experience of practical democracy, for example, some refugees, asylum seekers, migrant populations and political groups may also be disadvantaged. Others may not trust the democratic process or perceive public organisations as taking a persecutory or pejorative stance against them.

Patient and public involvement in health services relies for its legitimacy on engaging local people with their local health service; in part, this, like voting is an aspect of active citizenship. While involvement does not yield democratic accountability those who are involved are usually citizens and are seeking a form of accountability and responsiveness that is different from the ballot box. Giving citizens a chance to have a say in shaping health services is one of the key ways that government can respond to the electorate and particularly in an area of the public sphere that lacks more direct forms of democratic accountability.

Citizenship – taxpayers fund public health services

A second justification for greater patient and public involvement relates to the publicly funded nature of national health services. Emerging from a decade of public sector reform inspired by neo-liberal ideology, the current governments in OECD countries are still concerned with providing 'value for money' justifications for public spending. Further, as health services are publicly funded, there is widespread pressure to provide a greater public voice in decisions about the organisation and delivery of health services this is increasingly being tied to localism and responsiveness. Such an approach echoes the call of 'new managerialism' championed by Osborne and Gaebler (1992) and underpinning *Reinventing Government* in the United States. More recent reforms continue to embrace this philosophy by seeking to empower local front line staff to be more responsive to the expressed needs of service users; an approach apparent in recent UK health policy such as *Shifting the Balance of Power within the NHS* (Department of Health 2001a).

It is worth noting that most residents who are not citizens are taxpayers and potential patients. Under European Union (EU) legislation citizens of any Member State have a right to healthcare and other public sector services in any Member State (Richards 1999; Rosenmöller, McKee and Baeten 2006). There is growing convergence across EU countries for the need to tighten the qualification for access to health services particularly in light of the recent EU expansion. Media representations of the impact of health immigrants on an already strained health service pressures health providers to evaluate the legitimacy of patient entitlement on the basis of citizenship and country of residence. Such representations of the situation only add to increasing popular resistance in relation to access to healthcare for 'foreigners'.

The issue of entitlement and patient mobility has been central to current development of a European Commission draft directive published in July

2008 as *The Directive of the European Parliament for the Application of Cross-Border Healthcare Patients Rights.* Summing up the issue, EU Health Commissioner Markos Kyprianu said:

> The healthcare that patients need is sometimes best provided in another EU country . . . The European Court of Justice has ruled that patients have rights to cross-border care under Community law, but there are uncertainties about what this means in practice. A clear, practical framework is needed to enable patients and those who pay for, provide and regulate health services to take advantage of cross-border healthcare where that is the best solution. This will also help to unlock huge potential for European cooperation to help improve efficiency and effectiveness of all EU health systems, whilst respecting national responsibility for their organisation and financing.
>
> (eGov Monitor 2006)

We propose the term social citizenship to differentiate actions that illustrate the relationship between individuals in a population and the local institutions of that country from citizenship as applied in the more restrictive, technical sense by politicians and civil servants. User, public and patient involvement is better conceptualised in relation to social citizenship with the effectiveness of the relationship reflecting the degree to which particular localities and NHS organisations are passive or pro-active.

The term 'citizen' is problematic in discussions of patient and public involvement. To a great extent it serves as a catch-all for any individual resident in a community that seeks to have a voice but may reinforce tensions between members of a settled community and visitors, immigrants and refugees. There is no attempt to differentiate this category in terms of its different sources of power or legitimacy. While there is an acceptance that the category is not homogeneous, diversity is considered primarily in terms of formally defined disability, socioeconomic status and ethnicity. The recognition of the multiple sources of power of users, and the dependence of decision makers on user support, redraws the context within which conflict over the ability to influence decisions is played out. It also demonstrates the multi-layered aims of such interactions and processes.

Consumerism – informed consent

The shift from patient to customer, user or consumer has been central to the neo-liberal framework used to rationalise health services and promoted by both greater managerialism and marketisation. Such reforms have been buttressed by the promotion of greater patient choice and have sought to redefine, particularly in the minds of policy makers, the provision of health services to businesses selling healthcare. To be consumers, patients must have the necessary information to choose and their choices must have an impact on those who provide the services. Patient and public involvement is typified not as a partnership generating a dialogue and shared decision making but rather the collection of information from service users as the feedback mechanism and expression of consumer views, therefore creating one of the key prerequisites for market relationships.

Health policy across Europe has steadily moved towards the creation of market relationships and often has been led by British innovation.

> In contemporary Britain, citizenship is confused with consumerism and democracy with marketing. Choice and individualism are elevated to the status of moral imperatives . . . . The consumer is characterised not only by the right to choice but also by entitlement to redress.
>
> (Marinker 1996: 13)

Justifications and definitions of user involvement in public services range along a continuum between democratic and consumerist models (Croft and Beresford 1993; 1995; Feldberg and Vipond 1999). Typically, the distinctions relate to rights inherent in citizenship versus those of individual choice in the marketplace. As Ignatieff has asserted:

> It is a symptom of the crisis of citizenship . . . that most political rhetoric, whether left or right, addresses the electorate not as citizens but as taxpayers or as consumers. It is as if the market were determining the very language of political community.
>
> (Ignatieff 1995: 71)

The aim of user involvement and the methods used to engage users can only be understood in relation to the relative primacy of one or other of these justifications.

The evolution of an international patient and public involvement agenda

An attention to patient and public involvement has a long history and can be traced to the World Health Organisation's (WHO) *Declaration of Alma-Ata* that explicitly placed involvement on the international public health agenda: 'The people have the right and duty to participate individually and collectively in the planning and implementation of their healthcare' (WHO/UNICEF 1978a: Clause IV).

The emergence of the New Public Health (NPH) philosophy (Ashton and Seymour 1988; Goroya and Scambler 1998) suggests a more holistic approach emphasising both individual and collective action to address the underlying causes of poor health, and rehearses the benefits of enhanced participation discussed in the *Declaration of Alma-Ata* (1978). The generalised concepts that underpinned NPH are broad-based and therefore support for the philosophy draws on broad political spectrum and a range of different national perspectives (Baggott 2000).

This shift was emphasised in further documents published by the WHO. The *Ottawa Charter for Health Promotion* (WHO 1986) emphasised the role of empowerment in health promotion, and acknowledged the 'voice' of the community as an essential component in matters of health, living conditions and wellbeing. The *Sundsvall Statement on Supportive Environments for Health* (WHO 1991) suggested that empowerment of people and community participation were essential factors in the development of a sustainable and democratic health promotion approach. An emphasis on the importance of patients' rights is also apparent in *The Declaration on the Promotion of Patients' Rights in Europe* (WHO Regional Office Europe 1994).

These documents together with attention to significant change in health systems globally set the scene for the 'Ljubljana Charter on Reforming Health Care' which articulates a set of healthcare principles:

> Healthcare reforms must address citizens' needs, taking into account their expectations about health and healthcare. They should ensure that citizen's voice and choice decisively influence the way in which health services are designed and operate.
> (WHO Regional Office Europe 1996: Clause 5.3; see especially Clause 6.2)

The Ljubljana Charter was echoed by the Council of Europe (2000) and the programme of European Union action in the field of public health. This programme refers to 'visibility and transparency', information provision, and reinforces the notion of balance and proportionality in the context of public consultation and stakeholder participation in health protection involvement processes, noting that all health-related activities of the Community must incorporate a set of key elements.

> To contribute to the wellbeing of European citizens, the Community must address in a coordinated and coherent way the concerns of its people about risks to health and their expectations for a high level of health protection. Therefore, all health-related activities of the Community must have a high degree of visibility and transparency and allow consultation and participation of all stakeholders in a balanced way, in order to promote better knowledge and communication flows and thus enable a greater involvement of individuals in decisions that concern their health.
> (EU 2002: Article 1)

The trend towards greater citizen participation in state regulation of public goods and in particular the right to access relevant information was central to the ratification of the Aarhus Convention (United Nations Economic Commission for Europe 1998) by the European Union (EU 2005). This

Convention established a number of public rights concerning access to environmental information, the right to participate in environmental decision
making, the right to review procedures to challenge public decisions that have
been made without respecting the two aforementioned rights or environmental law in general. Although these provisions concern 'the environment', the
potential reach of the document is far greater. Critical to this is the acceptance
of the role of the public in the decision-making process.

The core health policy objective of the 2006 Finnish EU Presidency was to
promote the principle of *Health in All Policies*. The rationale for this formulation emphasises the understanding that good health is largely determined
by factors outside the domain of healthcare and policies other than health
have direct effects on health determinants. Such an approach contributes to
horizontal EU policy including the Lisbon Strategy. The *Health in All Policies*
agenda promotes patient and public involvement within the EU and reinforces the need for systematic evaluation of the implications of policies
and the use of the Health Impact Assessment methodology (HIA). The
Gothenburg Consensus Paper dealt with the values underpinning the implementation of Health Impact Assessment (HIA), emphasising 'The right of
people to participate in a transparent process for the formulation, implementation and evaluation of policies that affect their life, both directly and
through the elected political decision makers' (European Centre for Health
Policy and WHO Regional Office for Europe 1999: 4).

Other EU documents have emphasised the importance of the values-based
principle of 'participation in the decision-making process by those who may
be affected' (Stahl *et al.* 2006: 146) and the role of health impact assessment
as an integral part of this agenda as it incorporates aspects of public involvement.

The importance of collective capacity-building in local communities
and voluntary organisations, and organisational rather than individual
involvement embedded within civil society, is emphasised by the European
Commission: 'It is necessary to build up the organisations representing
patients and those developing the public health agenda so that civil society is
able to make the constructive contribution needed to public health policy'
(European Commission 2006a: 47).

The trend towards greater centrality of patient and public involvement
globally is clearly apparent and this is even more explicit within Europe.
International organisations such as the WHO have played a central role in
creating and documenting consensus around aspirations, principles and
rights that reinforce patient and public involvement in individual treatment
decisions, policy making and service development.

Policies that have promoted patient and public involvement

The degree of user involvement in other OECD countries varies but it seems
independent of the role or the nature of the health system. Developments in

the Netherlands, for example, have been more systematic, with a greater emphasis on legislation than those in the UK (Vos 2002). Denmark, like the other Nordic countries, involves patients and the public in the running of the health service through local democracy. In addition to the patients' rights and complaints systems that exist in most Nordic countries, patient organisations contribute actively to health service development and debate. By comparison, in Sweden and Finland, patient and public involvement is more passive and largely exercised through local elections. Despite the long history of acclaiming the importance of user involvement in Canadian health services, representing them as a continuum rather than a ladder, the legitimacy of many exercises continues to be challenged. Current structures are similar to those in England with an emphasis on competent citizen governors, public reporting of performance and various mechanisms to ensure that patients can access care and have their complaints addressed. The Romanow commission (2002) proposed developing citizen involvement in the policy development process and strengthening accountability between citizens and policy makers. Insufficient political will and tensions between national and territorial governments have blocked implementation.

Rather than the structure of the healthcare system (see Chapter 2) the nature of national law and policy has significant implications for the emergence and development of patient and public involvement. Typically, law takes two forms: rights-based or regulatory. A range of countries have enacted rights legislation that explicitly define patient rights or indirectly do so within the broader context of human rights. In 1992 Finland passed what it claimed was the first law specifically on patients' rights – The Act on the Status and Rights of Patients (785/1992). In 1994 the WHO Regional Office for Europe hosted a European Consultation on the Rights of Patients in Amsterdam. Drawing a distinction between individual patient rights and the responsibilities of the state to residents, social patient rights, the final report suggests:

> Social rights in healthcare relate to the societal obligation undertaken or otherwise enforced by government and other public or private bodies to make reasonable provision of healthcare for the whole population . . . . Social rights also relate to equal access to healthcare for all those living in a country or other geopolitical area and the elimination of unjustified discriminatory barriers, whether financial, geographical, cultural or social and psychological.
>
> (WHO Regional Office for Europe 1994: 6)

Most legislation when discussing patients' rights, frames them in terms of individual rights:

> Individual rights in patient care are more readily expressed in absolute terms and when made operational can be made enforceable on behalf of

an individual patient. These rights cover such areas as the integrity of the person, privacy and religious convictions.

(WHO Regional Office for Europe 1994: 6)

The alternative approach to safeguarding opportunities for patients to access health services in a just and equitable manner makes use of regulatory power. The United Kingdom, for instance, relies on formal regulators such as the Care Quality Commission and the National Institute for Health and Clinical Excellence, and statutory instruments to direct healthcare providers to achieve these goals.

These different approaches imply a primacy of the individual in countries adopting a patient rights model and the embracing of collectivism in those countries utilising a regulatory approach. Further, that this would also be reflected in orientations to key policies such as 'patient choice' that promotes individual level action in the pursuit of individual health benefits. Sweden, for instance, has long been pursuing a patient choice agenda since 2003 (Swedish Institute 2003). The implementation has accelerated significantly since the election of the Moderate Party led alliance in 2006 (a conservative led agenda of privatisation of health services).

Ironically, it is in the United Kingdom that a high profile focus on patient choice has been readily apparent since 2003 (Department of Health 2003a; 2003c; 2004b; 2006c). In implementation terms, individual patient choice is very varied and dependent on information primarily provided through the internet. The *Choose and Book* service enables patients at registered General Practices who are referred for secondary investigations and treatments to choose the location where the intervention will be delivered. Since 2008, patients can choose any acute NHS hospital across England and also a number of private institutions.

To enable patient choice, information is provided on the distance to the hospital, travel and parking arrangements, appointment times and the rating of the hospital by the Healthcare Commission on a four point scale: poor, adequate, good and excellent. Some additional information may be available through the *NHS Choices* website. That is the choice is almost solely based on location. There is no scope to specify the physician or the particular intervention (e.g. type of surgical procedure).

These different frameworks within which patient choice must be articulated have consequences for patient and public involvement. A rights-based approach often builds on existing human rights legislation or treaties, and frames appropriate access to services as an individual entitlement. Associated with this entitlement are the consequential requirements for access to information and justice without which competition would not be possible. In contrast a regulatory approach places requirements on those who plan, fund and provide health services.

For a regulatory approach, patient and public involvement can be integrated into the requirements around planning, evaluation and delivery of services. Patients and the public can be involved in the training and appointment of healthcare professionals and the generation of evidence (involvement in research). For a rights-based approach it is far more difficult to require involvement in processes of planning and delivery as patient involvement is defined as the active, conscious choosing of some services over others. From this perspective public involvement is simply the aggregation of individual decisions. This distinction in the framing of the nature and role of patient and public involvement suggests different conceptions of the relationship between the state and the citizen. Similarly, *the public* is a category not a collective.

Patient and public involvement has emerged on the health policy scene as a response to a series of tensions – individual/collective; consumerism/patient-centred; rights/regulation – and is being adopted for diverse reasons from cost-containment and shifting responsibility to better tailoring of services to meet the needs of patients and communities. Despite this contestation of ends patient and public involvement holds the potential to redraw not only the relationship between those who provide healthcare and those who use these services but the culture of health services and the position and responsibility of the state.

2 Health policies, health systems and healthcare reforms

The context of health policies and health systems is changing. Our understanding of health policy priorities as well as the tasks and functions that health systems are to take are based on values, evidence and political compromise. More fundamentally, judgments about the appropriate functions of health systems and the legitimate aims of health policies shape our understanding. These set the framework for the analysis of healthcare reforms as well as interface of public participation and healthcare reforms.

What are health systems and their priorities?

Health policies are part of normative policy making within a society, and are therefore embedded in the legal rights and commitments made as part of public policies. Health policies are typically based on values, evidence, experience, knowledge and technical expertise. Health systems can be seen as the institutional expression of health policies. Health systems thus cover more than health services for individuals (Mackintosh and Koivusalo 2005).

The World Health Organisation Regional Office for Europe (WHO/Europe) definition of health systems maintains both the health and social security aspects of health systems:

> The people, institutions and resources, arranged together in accordance with established policies, to improve the health of the population they serve, while responding to people's legitimate expectations and protecting them against the cost of ill-health through a variety of activities whose primary intent is to improve health.
>
> (WHO Regional Office for Europe 2000)

Health systems include functions for which health is the first priority and are essentially population based, including public health, health promotion and assessment of health implications of other policies. As the legitimacy of health systems is derived from political commitments made to citizens by the government, the accountability and responsibility for their proper functioning lie in the public domain and cannot be left solely to consumer choice and action.

Crucially, the organisation and functioning of health systems are grounded and constrained by the culture, resources, and values of a country, yet operate in a field of medical care and normative policies which is open to international exchange and learning (Mackintosh and Koivusalo 2005).

If health systems are considered in this context and as a means to achieve health policy aims, common technical issues between countries become more evident. However, health systems are also essential in the context of social security, trust and social cohesion in the society. Health systems are also recognised as mechanisms and means for distribution and redistribution of resources. One essential aspect of health systems is the way in which these address solidarity and equity in terms of cross-subsidising between those who are healthy and ill as well as across rich and poor people and areas. This aspect of health systems has become increasingly important in the context of health financing and the organisation of healthcare and as part of a broader concern with the equity and solidarity aspects of health systems.

Health systems have become less clearly defined with an overemphasis on health services and the managerial aspects of health systems and less on what they actually are set out to achieve. This has encouraged a tendency to focus on health status or outcomes as measure of health system functioning. However, health systems can be addressed more in terms of what these are supposed to do. Mackintosh and Koivusalo have defined these tasks as the following (Mackintosh and Koivusalo 2005):

1   protection and promotion of population health and provision of preventive services, inter-sectoral action and emergency preparedness ('public health')
2   provision of health services and care for all according to need, and financing it according to ability to pay ('health services')
3   ensuring training, surveillance and research for the maintenance and improvement of population health and health services and availability of a skilled labour force ('human resources and knowledge')
4   ensuring ethical integrity and professionalism, mechanism of policy development, planning and accountability, citizen rights, participation and involvement of users and respect of confidentiality and dignity in provision of services ('ethics, accountability and policy').

It is in this context that healthcare reforms and their implications need to be assessed and evaluated against health policy priorities and aims. It is also in this context that governments need to address their capacities for ensuring sufficient policy space for implementing health policies that cannot be seen merely as another commercial sector responding to consumer wants.

Globalisation and healthcare: incentives and pressures

The impact of globalisation on health systems is mediated by national policy priorities and practices, including the ways in which governments wish to prioritise health and health policy aims in comparison to other priorities. Both power sharing between global and national actors, and more importantly how globalisation processes empower and mediate power relations and change across sectors within countries, shape the impact of globalisation. We have defined globalisation as the process of global economic integration, which is moulded by technological change, but not a requirement of it. We also wish to draw attention to the importance of the politics of globalisation and the implicit assumptions of what implications globalisation is to have upon health systems or their reform. It is in this context that five trends of globalisation influence the articulation of health policy.

1   The requirement to lower costs due to pressures of *global competitiveness*. Global economic competitiveness arguments are used in the context of expectations and assumptions that call for limiting the funding of social security systems at the chosen levels and to limiting the overall size of the public sector workforce. This is also reflected in the European Union focus on public budgets and concerns over healthcare costs in the light of pressures due to aging (Council of Europe 2004). Low public spending on health, which has previously been framed as a value is now articulated more as a necessity. In countries with larger public sector workforce, moves towards a more contractual and competitive bidding to deliver services have also been articulated as means for limiting the size of welfare states in the light of future demographic change.

2   The emergence of *innovation* as means to tackle global competitiveness has become more clearly articulated in many countries, and within the European Union. This is important for three distinct reasons. First, innovation is usually perceived to need greater private and commercial sector engagement. Second, innovation tends to lead to an emphasis on new product, concept and practice development in comparison to their evaluation and assessment. Third, innovation creates cost and access pressures within the health sector. New technologies and pharmaceuticals are often priced markedly higher due to the incentive structures for pharmaceutical research legitimised on the basis of supporting innovation. Doran and Henry (2008) have pointed out how innovation needs were used as a means to change the scope of national pharmaceutical policies and the use of price control mechanisms. The needs for innovation were, for example, also raised by proponents of the pharmaceutical industry in Finland in the context of the shift towards reference pricing in pharmaceuticals (Lääketeollisuus 2008).

3   The changing *power relations between different sectors* within societies and within governments. A focus on export markets for services emphasises the commercial potential of health services as part of tradable services both within the European Union as well as internationally, and emphasises the requirements to provide market access to other service providers. Health systems become important due to their

commercial potential and their performance is evaluated in this context. The purpose of health systems shifts from existing health policy priorities to the scope for commercial success. National policies then become more responsive to the interests of commercial providers and as part of trade and industrial policies. Globalisation also opens up scope for increasing consideration of health systems as a *resource base, payer and growing ground* for globalising industries and their needs. This is reflected in attention to e-health, telemedicine and advanced medical technologies. These technologies require major resource shifts within health systems as do other areas such as biotechnology, genetic tests and new medicines. Health systems in this context are not intrinsically important but considered fertile ground for other industries to develop.

4   Globalisation arguments are also used to empower models and means of health systems provision and financing that allow for the mobility and portability of benefits required by globalisation. This leads to a stress on *individual mobility* and has significant implications for the models of healthcare organisation and financing. This articulation is present both in the general assessment of globalisation in terms of enabling mobility and migration as well as, for example, in the context of European policies and issues with respect to patient mobility, internal markets and health. At the global level migration becomes the means to cover needs for health professionals. However, while developed countries and in particular the United Kingdom and the United States have been the winners in health professionals' migration, the situation in many countries is increasingly worrying due to the consequential lack of workforce (Buchan and Sochalski 2004; Diallo 2004; Stillwell *et al.* 2004; Narashiman *et al.* 2003; Saravia and Miranda 2004; Mensah 2005).

5   Finally, *taking intergovernmental regulatory frameworks as given* rather than negotiated outcomes undermining or overstating their implications upon available *national policy space for health*. International agreements affect the ways in which national policies can be implemented as well as serve as the basis for incentives for research and development, sharing of data and access to knowledge, but too strong an emphasis on their importance also limits potential policy space. The interface between national, European and global policies is not always clear or explicit, but there is a danger that *existing international agreements and commitments are interpreted as inflexible or unchangeable,* even when these might have detrimental impacts upon health systems across different countries. A case in point can be made with respect to the relationship between internal markets and health policies within European Union.

The politics of globalisation is important to the ways in which health systems are reformed in order to respond to the pressures and needs which globalisation necessitates; more often reforms are premised on the assumed requirements of globalisation (see Chapters 4 and 5).

Healthcare reforms

The term healthcare reform does not imply any particular change in health services, but has become associated with policies with a particular set of changes in the organisation, financing and management of health services. Healthcare reforms as a concept has a particular reference to a specific type of reform initiated in the 1980s as part of a set of new public management oriented public sector reforms in many countries. One of the essential elements of these reforms was an assumption that governments should steer, but not row (Osborne and Gaebler 1992), thus encouraging a split between the purchaser and the provider functions of health services and a shift to the reliance on explicit contractual relationships.

Another important element in healthcare reforms has been the use of competition, choice and market forces, typically framed in terms of managed competition and articulated by its main proponent Alain Enthoven (see Enthoven 1993; OECD 1992). The Enthoven reform proposals, initially designed for America where *socialised medicine* could not be approved (Waitzkin 1994), diffused more strongly to the United Kingdom and other European countries, such as the Netherlands and Sweden (Maynard and Bloor 1995; Ham and Brommels 1994; Blomqvist 2002).

In terms of globalisation, healthcare reforms have been part of the agenda of global institutions and policy making since the late 1980s, when an analysis of healthcare reforms was initiated within the Organisation for Economic Co-operation and Development (OECD). This was in part an independent process, but ran parallel to a more general focus on public sector reforms and the promotion of the principles and practice of new public management in the context of public services. While new public management has been promoted as a 'global transformation' (see Kettl 2000), the ways in which countries have or have not embarked on reform changes or how international agencies have become proponents of this change has been important for their diffusion.

The relevance of the OECD in the context of articulating healthcare reform has been important for the globalisation of the ideas and practice of healthcare reforms, even though the organisation does not have enforcement capacities (Moran and Wood 1996). Other processes of globalisation can be found in the content and politics of international health policies and the relative shifts from the dominant position of the WHO and the *Health for All* strategy to an era of healthcare reforms influenced to a large extent by the World Bank (Koivusalo and Ollila 1997). Lee and Goodman have brought up the importance of epistemic networks in providing the framework and production of knowledge on the basis of which broader policies were initiated and implemented (see Lee and Goodman 2002). In this context the OECD and the professional networks of (health) economists can be seen as part of an epistemic network promoting healthcare and public sector reform within Europe. An academic and comparative interest in healthcare reforms clearly resided in the OECD during the early 1990s (OECD 1992; OECD 1996; Oxley and Macfarlan 1995).

The WHO undertook a broad review on healthcare reform processes with a more critical overview and emphasis as part of the Ljubljana Conference and Charter. The 'Ljubljana Charter on Reforming Health Care', however, both took on board some of the managerial issues as well as critically raised equity, universal access and other concerns on the basis of 'sound financing' arguments (WHO 1996). The promotion and diffusion of ideas and emphasis of healthcare reforms internationally can be seen in the context of both healthcare reform related language and as part of a broader set of regulatory reforms and pressures to modernise health systems. The former has been articulated in the context of OECD work and this emphasis is reflected later in, for example, European emphasis on modernisation (see Chapter 5).

In this chapter we reflect on our findings on healthcare reforms in the light of the early predictions by Dahlgren (1990), suggesting that the initial healthcare reforms were only the first stage of the commercialisation process. Our interest in healthcare reforms is in understanding the extent to which the initial healthcare reforms efforts aimed at lowering costs have shifted their focus. That is, have healthcare reforms rather than focusing on cost-containment become the mechanism for greater outsourcing, choice and use of market mechanisms in publicly funded services with less consideration of overall resource use? We then ask to what extent there could be a further shift towards a third stage of reforms with more commercialised and individualised context of financing of services as well.

The first phase of healthcare reforms

The initial phase of healthcare reforms in OECD countries was based on ideas that emphasised the use of competition and market mechanisms in the context of health services provision with the assumption that this would lead towards lower costs and improved efficiency. The first phase of European and OECD member state experiences in healthcare reforms have been extensively discussed and assessed (see e.g. OECD 1995; 2003a; Maynard and Bloor 1995; Saltman and Figueiras 1997; European Health Management Association 2000; Cabiedes and Guillen 2001).

In Europe the initial *reformers* were the United Kingdom, the Netherlands and Sweden (Ham and Brommels 1994). The reform model in this *first phase* was influenced by concepts of planned markets and managed competition within the public sector or within formal statutory social security systems. This thinking was influenced to a large extent by broader principles of new public management as the means to improve the public sector, and within the health sector the application of managed competition/public competition or internal markets as means to implement the reforms.

The OECD health project account of healthcare reforms was, however, critical in terms of the extent to which the use of competitive mechanisms can deliver the expected gains and in relation to the importance of ensuring cross-subsidisation (Docteur and Oxley 2003). The lack of evidence of benefits from competition led to waning enthusiasm for the initial healthcare reform processes within OECD countries.

The lack of political success of the first phase of healthcare reforms can partly be explained by changes in politics. In many countries, including the United Kingdom, Sweden and Finland the predominantly social democratic governments did not fully abolish the organisational structures created under more conservative governments but in contrast allowed them to expand. The political process of healthcare reforms in Nordic countries is best understood in the context of further reforms undertaken by more right-wing governments and local councils, which do not fully revert after changes in power. In England under a new Labour government these moves were recognised by Enthoven himself who noted, 'I find it a great irony that a British Labour government appears to be well ahead of private-sector employer-purchasers in the USA when it comes to bringing market forces to bear on healthcare services' (Enthoven 2002).

The lessons from the first phase of health reform were not only about the limits of market-based reforms in reducing costs, but also the increased administrative costs associated with the managerial restructuring of the service provision and administration.

Commercialisation and the first phase of healthcare reforms

It can be claimed that the first phase of healthcare reforms was undertaken as a process of commercialising principles of operation within public services in order to reduce costs, or in the case of Sweden to also limit professional power and enhance accountability. The resulting changes created organisational structures and processes which were more amenable to further commercialisation, but the first phase of healthcare reforms delivered relatively few opportunities and only limited focus for commercialisation more broadly.

However, what the first phase of reform did achieve was to create the legal and organisational structures required to enable markets in publicly funded service provision. It thus changed the organisation and the context in which services were provided and regulated. The creation of a purchaser–provider split was crucial for the further commercialisation of health systems. The first phase of health reforms also led to the establishment of a new type of commercial operator that focused on publicly funded service provision markets. One example of this type of commercial operator is the Swedish Capio, which has had a particular interest in the contractual markets of public services (Lethbridge 2005).

Another aspect of the first stage reform process has taken place in the context of creating a *level playing field*. The introduction of Diagnostic Related Groups (DRGs) within health systems provides the scope for further engagement with the private sector in the delivery of services (Lethbridge 2005).

DRG categories allow providers to calculate average cost for different types of health interventions and commissioners to set maximum prices for reimbursement. In terms of contracting out and implementing health reforms, DRGs can be seen as an intermediary step towards engaging more fully with private sector actors as part of provider organisations. Governments are thus no longer as necessary as direct providers of services, but rather as the financiers and regulators of service provision.

The first phase of health reforms were driven by the aim of controlling of costs and reorganising the supply side and thus provided little opportunity for patients, citizens or service users to shape or influence the process. However, the ability of market oriented measures to control the costs of healthcare appears also to have been less successful than the *command and control* systems they replaced. The disenchantment with healthcare reforms was also mediated through government changes. For example, in Sweden the social democratic government introduced the so called *stop-law*, which limited the opportunities to sell public hospitals (Glenngård *et al.* 2005).

The second phase of healthcare reforms

The second phase of healthcare reforms arose at the end of 1990s in Sweden (Harrison and Callthorp 2000). However, in contrast with the first phase of reforms, the second phase has been less systemic and mostly driven by operators and actors outside the health service. It could in many ways be considered an incremental process rather than a radical redesign. While the first phase of reforms created the legal structures and shifted power to managerial positions within the public sector, the second phase of reforms are promoted in particular from outside the sector and by national and European actors who champion competition and contracting out.

Ideologically the second phase of reforms is likely to be driven less by the requirement of actually reducing financial burden of the health system and more on the basis of considering the health sector and services as a commercial sector providing jobs, productivity and export potential. Further, this has had an added impetus through the reconceptualising of the health system as a support for industrial approaches to innovation and knowledge products in biotechnology and pharmaceuticals. This approach can be seen at present in the context of the recent arguments on trade in health services, internal markets and pharmaceutical policies (Mattoo and Rathindran 2006; European Commission 2003). Mattoo and Rathindran (2006) in a United States context ask whether healthcare is so different from other goods that it cannot be regarded as tradable. They consider the reasons for the *underuse* of overseas services in the context of US policies could be due to implicit protection for domestic providers or the oligopolistic nature of the health insurance industry and thus the lack of competition.

The pressure for change and increased productivity that is taking place as part of the second phase of health reforms emerges from the market-based regulatory aims and actors. Health systems are no longer important primarily because they ensure that people gain access to health services when in need and irrespective of their ability to pay, that epidemics are prevented or controlled or health outcomes improved due to health promotion efforts or that the social determinants of health are addressed as part of public policies. In the emerging context of the reform policies, health systems are important not only as providers of products and services for which people are willing to pay, but also as an investment opportunity within global financial markets.

It is in this context that the articulation of the purpose of health systems on the one hand, and the extension of commercial policy mechanisms to the ways in which health systems are financed, organised and managed on the other, become of importance. As the structures in healthcare organisation and management have been reformed to fit the services trade it is now possible to implement rules and regulatory measures that create greater scope for trade in healthcare and services. The structural change in services has now enabled the enhancement of contracting out to the private sector companies and requirements for doing so can be enforced, in a European context, through broader commitments to internal markets and government procurement (see Chapter 5).

In contrast to the *supply-side* focus of first phase of health reforms the new focus in the second phase is shifting to the *demand-side*, emphasising consumer as patients and granting them rights to choose their service provider. In contrast to the earlier emphasis on costs and cost-cutting the emphasis is now on choice and quality of services; as choice emerges as a key aspect of the health reform process it requires changes to existing health policy priorities. The purpose of market mechanisms and strategies is now no longer to ensure lower costs, but rather to ensure quality and innovation.

The emphasis on individual consumer choice can be seen as the means and basis on which there is scope for creating a plurality of providers and has become part of a broader agenda for reform within health systems. The emphasis on patient choice as part of healthcare reform becomes a means of service improvement and in practice a mechanism that legitimates the creation of markets, the inclusion of a plurality of non public providers and greater opportunity for the providers to choose their patients.

Commercialisation and the second phase of healthcare reforms

The role of commercialisation in the second phase of healthcare reforms is most evident in the transformation from being a mechanism for cost-containment to a mechanism to satisfy requirements for patient choice. This phase of reform enhances the prospects for commercial gains and productivity of the private sector and reframes the aim of health system as contributor to the economy and location for future business prospects in the underdeveloped services and export sector. In this context and articulation markets, competition and choice are intended to deliver ultimately the best possible system, and commercialisation becomes an end rather than a means for improvement. However, in the current context of publicly financed services, the main scope for commercialisation remains in the provision of publicly funded services.

The level of commercialisation brought about by the second phase of health reforms and the adjustment to a more market-based regulatory environment is likely to remain the situation for publicly provided services. Until cost-containment and regulatory interference become more significant there is little scope for a possible third phase of reforms in the financing of healthcare. However, in many ways most European countries remain between first and second stages, having implemented a structural purchaser–provider split but with only limited choice and private sector engagement in the provision of healthcare services.

The prospects of a third phase of reform

The third phase of healthcare reforms of the financing of healthcare can be envisaged, although it is in many ways still to emerge. The expected orientation of this phase of reforms, should the direction remain the same, would be towards financing models that increase private spending on health in order to secure public spending for poorer sections of society.

The promotion of patient choice of provider of services creates the basis for shifting to a choice of health plans or different forms of financing. Such a shift creates the framework and incentive structure for not only greater and more diverse forms of co-payment but the purchasing of additional access or scope of services directly or in the form of more personalised insurance and for 'consumer driven' models of healthcare.

As a result of this process three types of incremental shift are likely. First, moving towards a private insurance-based system, where public funding or insurance covers those who are otherwise uninsurable. Second, the move towards individual health saving accounts with insurance to cover acute care costs. Third, patching together diverse arrangements on the basis of availability of resources. These could include employer-based private insurance schemes and any other schemes dependent upon consumer choice and eligibility and different publicly financed mechanisms to cover those who are not and will not be covered otherwise.

In the view of those promoting these changes, a low-level of public funding and high-level of consumer choice are envisaged providing both opportunities for commercial growth through increasing overall resources to health as well as lowering the overall share of public funding on health.

The idea of patient choice as a crucial *steering* mechanism for health system functioning creates the fundamental problem of sounding great in empowering patients as key actors at policy level, but becomes problematic in practice by creating overwhelming reliance on the nature and quality of choices that patients are willing and able to make. It is, in this context, necessary to pose the counter question in terms of the extent to which choice has worked as the steering mechanism in other areas, where traditional market failures such as information asymmetry are not as rife or products and services are more clearly defined than in health. The lure inherent in an emphasis on patient or consumer-driven healthcare needs should be critically assessed because of the potential scope for cost escalation as a result of choice.

The articulation of consumer-driven healthcare is part of the broader interest where individualisation of financial burden has been combined with incentives to healthier lifestyle and prevention as part of higher personal governance over costs of care. However, this type of emphasis on *financial responsibility incentives to choosing healthy lifestyle* approach, which can be seen as attractive to economists and policy makers, does ignore fundamental facts and known aspects in the causation of health and disease. While adjustments could be made with respect to diseases in exclusion of fully hereditary diseases or the rather large number of diseases and conditions for which causal pathways are not known, the moral dilemmas as well as the extent to which individuals are likely to be able to change their lifestyle or habits will remain a fundamental concern.

The reform of financing could enable further commercialisation of services as well as bring additional private funds to the sector, but individualised financing mechanisms are brought as additional rather than alternative mechanism. The groundwork for this type of reform is based on the creation of mechanisms through which payments and information follow the patients in the form of, for instance, health cards or portable electronic patient records. While a European health card with information following the patient could enable *free choice* within a European market, it is unlikely that it would in practice lead to significant take up of particular services from different providers (see Chapter 3). Other mechanisms for this are vouchers, which can be initially fully publicly funded and slowly decline in terms of their value and share of the costs of care.

Globalisation, healthcare and markets and national policy space

A striking concern in respect to many of the currently promoted initiatives concerning patient choice and competition as mechanisms for implementing healthcare reforms is the limited evidence of actual public demand. There is also little evidence that the changes proposed in the reforms actually deliver major improvements in terms of either cost-containment or choice. The evidence from the first stage of health reforms are at best mixed. The analysis of experiences and cross-country outcomes in the global context do not support the benefits of expanding commercialisation, but in contrast note the lack of benefits at the global level (Mackintosh and Koivusalo 2005).

The absence and limitations of the evidence base on competition and commercialisation in healthcare is recognised even in the context of the European Competitiveness Report in 2004 (European Commission 2004e). In OECD countries most evidence on competition seems to be derived from experiences in the USA and in particular California (Propper *et al.* 2005). However, the relevance of experiences in the USA to the very different way that health systems operate in Europe is contested.

Healthcare reforms are contested and the political context for individual countries limits the scope and basis for the implementation of the strategies we have outlined. This does not exclude, however, a process of incremental change through the inclusion of various mechanisms from internal market rules and government procurement stipulations to bilateral and multilateral trade agreements covering services and investments. Globalisation can be seen in this context both as a means for promoting healthcare reforms in order to lower public spending on healthcare, but also contributing to more commercialised and individualised solutions.

Health policies tend to be compared within national contexts and the recent emphasis on historical institutionalism as part of this comparison may not have given sufficient importance to the ways in which health systems may be reforming. The similarities become undermined by the differences in the nature and power of how various stakeholders shape, influence and exert pressure resulting in different policy articulation in each country (see Evans 2005). Reforms may also be promoted or have been promoted under different emphases and overarching claims relating to modernisation, demographic change, decentralisation, user choice, productivity or innovation.

While globalisation or the politics of globalisation and particular economic policy priorities can be identified at the core of the pressures for the second phase of healthcare reform, this does not imply that these changes are inevitable or desirable from a health policy perspective. Rather, one of the main points that we seek to make is that as pressures come from needs and priorities outside health systems and are based on assumptions made outside the health sector, these may not only limit the availability of resources for health but also the regulatory space that national health administrations have. National policy space is a term raised by developing countries in the context of trade policies, but it can be articulated as well with a focus on health policies as national policy space does not guarantee that this regulatory scope is used for the benefit of health or health policy priorities (see e.g. Koivusalo *et al.* 2009).

The claiming of a national policy space for health is important for governments if they are to remain accountable for the provision of health services to their citizens. In this context we observe that the aims of, and needs for, health policies in a national context differ. In other words, in order to make a case for national policies separate from commercial priorities an understanding of national health policy priorities, needs, aims and means must be explicit and clear. Health policies need to become understood as part of public policies and in relation to the values and aims of these policies. Health policy priorities need also to reach beyond a set of desired health outcomes as it matters how and through what means the desired outcomes are sought. In the light of agreements and policies designed to meet primarily commercial policy interests in international fora, there is a need to recognise better the crucial common interests in health policies and policy aims at European and global levels. Such commonalities are not only in traditional policies such as for communicable diseases, but also in safeguarding the scope to base national health policies on health and health policy priorities and the values and principles underpinning these policies. This has relevance in particular to the ways in which organisation and financing of health systems relates to collective risk and resource-sharing mechanisms within systems. It also has relevance for extent to which values and principles, such as universality, equity and solidarity and access to good quality care, can become realised within health systems.

3 From patients to consumers

Healthcare has historically been organised around the needs and convenience of the experts and assumed that patients would find their way to the place where clinical knowledge resides. This model of patients as supplicants and physicians doling out advice based on their expertise has been challenged by the growth of alternative and complementary medicine, and the acknowledgement of patient expertise particularly in relation to long-term conditions. A second set of challenges to this model has come from the state as a primary funder, and often employer, of health professionals, and as part of larger, often neo-liberal-inspired managerial reforms that have sought greater accountability. A third source of challenge to traditional models of medical hierarchy and control has emerged from the public as – citizens and taxpayers who have asserted the need for responsiveness to the views, expectations and needs of the population rather than those of government or clinical experts. Together these challenges have shifted traditional models of medical hierarchy and are redefining the meaning of patient-centred care through calls for greater involvement of patients in decisions about their own healthcare and public inclusion in the evaluation and development of health services and research as a way of shaping and prioritising the knowledge base.

These pressures are in tension as some seek to promote greater individual patient influence while others seek to promote collective power in shaping services and the national health agenda. This chapter explores these tensions and suggests that we are seeing continual attempts to frame the nature of the doctor–patient relationship and indeed the patient–health system relationship in market terms, where the patient is not the shaper of the priorities and agenda but rather a customer and consumer.

The involvement policy agenda

Patient and public involvement, whether framed as patient rights or regulatory requirements on publicly funded healthcare planners and providers, is now a central element of contemporary healthcare reform internationally (see Chapter 1). The foundation of patient and public involvement can be seen in the emergence of patient-centred healthcare in part as a response to a decade of evidence-based healthcare that had, arguably, constrained and limited medical power and dominance. Patient-centred care reframes the doctor–patient relationship, focuses attention on contextual decision making, and reinforces the centrality of physician as information provider and guide to treatment decisions. Although this shift in health policy has been apparent in Europe, it is also visible more broadly around the world (see, for instance, Health Canada 2000; Government of Western Australia 2006). This framework is supported by the increased focus on lay knowledge, patient experience and self-management, and promoted by initiatives such as the Expert Patient Programme (Department of Health 1999b; Chief Medical Officer 2006).

Patient-centred care is typically predicated on creating opportunities and responding to a patient's desire for information and participation in treatment decision making in a medical consultation. The evolution of patient-centred care has been broad-based, although the impact on either practice or patient experience has been mixed (Dale *et al.* 2008). As Stewart has observed:

> Patient centredness is becoming a widely used, but poorly understood, concept in medical practice. It may be most commonly understood for what it is not – technology centred, doctor centred, hospital centred, disease centred. Definitions of patient centred care seek to make the implicit in patient care explicit.
>
> (Stewart 2001: 444)

A second strand that has reinforced the emergence of patient and public involvement has been government rhetoric regarding the need to provide increased accountability to citizens and taxpayers. Together these justifications have generated a redefinition of 'patient-centred healthcare' that has led to increasing pressure to 'involve' patients in decisions about their own care, service evaluation, development and research.

Justifications and definitions of user involvement in public services range along a continuum between democratic and consumerist models (Croft and Beresford 1993; Feldberg and Vipond 1999). Typically, the distinctions relate to rights inherent in citizenship versus those of individual choice in the marketplace. As Ignatieff has asserted:

> It is a symptom of the crisis of citizenship . . . that most political rhetoric, whether left or right, addresses the electorate not as citizens but as taxpayers or as consumers. It is as if the market were determining the very language of political community.
>
> (Ignatieff 1995: 71)

Involvement as a central plank of healthcare policy is distinct from the neo-liberal inspired healthcare reforms that have been at the heart of structural change in health systems internationally since the 1990s. The pressure to promote local involvement as part of implicit and explicit policy is also driven by the patterned decentralisation of health services that is apparent across Europe. Market forces, however, continue to be the touchstone for healthcare reform. The reframing of a healthcare system that is predicated on services free at the point of delivery, which aim to limit inequality, has consequences not only for the definition of the patient and service user but also for governance and accountability to the public. The rhetoric of greater involvement of the public in shaping public services has been described as *mimic consumerism* (Klein 2001). In part this highlights the tensions between involvement and consumerism which are particularly apparent in relation to individual action.

Harnessing the power of markets: the role of patient choice

The patient choice agenda is reflected in health policies that present opportunities for patients, the direct recipients of treatment and care, to select between different locations, providers, health professionals, or type of intervention. Most policies focus on one element of choice and typically this is the location where an intervention will be delivered or the clinician responsible for the intervention. A classic example of the former is apparent in the approach taken by the English NHS in the *Choose and Book service*, while the latter is evident in the approach to primary care in Stockholm.

The NHS *Choose and Book service*

It is in the United Kingdom that a commitment to patient choice in health policy has been apparent since 2003 (Department of Health 2003a; 2003c; 2004b; 2006c). The highest profile and most obvious attempt to implement patient choice has been through the *Choose and Book service* that enables patients referred by their General Practitioner for secondary investigations and treatments to 'choose' between a minimum of four acute hospitals or clinics at least one of which will be private. From April 2008 this was expanded to include all NHS hospitals across England although not all primary care practices are part of the service. Supported by a dedicated *NHS Choices* website patients can identify and compare hospitals based on their distance from a home address, travel and parking arrangements and the most recent rating by the Healthcare Commission (poor, adequate, good or excellent). In some instances further information about available treatments, facilities and patient support and patient feedback is also available but in practice this is very limited and varied. Once the patient has determined their *choice* they call a special telephone number and seek to make an appointment or book 'online' through the *HealthSpace* website.

Choose and Book in a system like the NHS, where general practitioners are both service providers and purchasers of secondary services as practice-based commissioners (Department of Health 2004b), presents particular governance challenges. Many physicians have responded to this by distancing themselves from the process of patient choice. Here, the outcome of the doctor–patient interaction is not a decision but rather a letter to patients setting out the options and leaving them to telephone a service to enact their decision. In this sense, the practical outcome of the choice agenda is a slower process with less opportunity for patients to maximise relevant information at the appropriate point in their decision, and more limited opportunities for physicians to refer patients to named clinical staff.

State funded healthcare systems have a duty to ensure the equitable allocation of scarce resources in the context of increasing demand. In this sense, healthcare systems 'manage' expectations in context of scarce resources. However, although patient choice via patient-focused care in the context of informed consent claims to equalise power differentials between health experts and the community, the excess service capacity implicit in and necessary for choice implies greater costs as well as opportunities.

Types of patient choice

The evolution of consumerism in health policy is, in part, justified as promoting patient-focused care through driving performance, whilst remaining affordable within the constraints of a tax-funded system. Similarly, consumerism is presented as a mechanism for redressing the power inequality between health professionals and patients and as the logical extension of informed consent. The marketisation of healthcare is based on creating opportunities for alternative providers of healthcare and mechanisms for patients to choose between. Given that the exercise of choice is predicated on a surplus in supply, this points to an inherent inefficiency in such a health system. Such a system also requires readily available information to enable the consumer, or those purchasing on their behalf, to choose.

There are different types of patient choice set at different levels of the health system. At the base level, patient choice is about the choice of healthcare professional responsible for delivering care. This is different, but often linked, to choice of specific treatments; different clinical staff have experience or a propensity for some treatments rather than others. For instance, some doctors are willing to countenance complementary therapies as part of a treatment regimen for cancer while others refuse to integrate these into the care programme for which they are responsible. Of course, proximity or travelling may be required to access a chosen healthcare professional (Exworthy and Peckham 2006), and the doctor may not choose to take on all of the patients who approach them.

At an organisational level, choice can be exercised between different healthcare settings; the organisational context within which care is organised, managed and delivered. Choice may be limited to public sector organisations or include private or non-profit organisations as well. However, as marketisation of healthcare systems has progressed, the distinctions between these different organisations are less clear. In a contract-driven model of publicly financed healthcare, the funding may remain public but the staff and organisations who deliver care are increasingly likely to be from the private or non-profit sector.

For many health systems choice is defined as a decision of which health plan (see Zalmanov 1997), health insurer, or health maintenance organisation to choose (Henke and Schreyögg 2004; Altenstetter and Busse 2005). Despite this being framed as choice, in practice, once a plan is specified, potential providers are defined by the plan and choice is more tightly constrained. Whatever plan is chosen, it will limit the choice of providers by requiring either authorisation or provision from a plan's network. In this context, preferred provider organisations and point of service organisations use financial incentives to constrain patient choice of provider (Docteur *et al.* 2003).

A new model of healthcare, tied to a rhetoric of patient choice is particularly apparent in the United States, where personal health accounts seek to address some of the constraints apparent in health insurance and health maintenance organisations. Presented as much as a tax-free investment vehicle, medical savings accounts, health reimbursement accounts and flexible spending accounts all provide incentives for *spending* less on healthcare. As the United States Treasury explains:

> A Health Savings Account is an alternative to traditional health insurance; it is a savings product that offers a different way for consumers to pay for their healthcare. HSAs (Health Savings Accounts) enable you to pay for current health expenses and save for future qualified medical and retiree health expenses on a tax-free basis.
>
> (US Department of the Treasury 2008)

All of these different approaches to providing patient choice are constrained. Some constraints relate to patient's resources (both information or financial), while others are associated with proximity and availability. Here, since further constraints may be defined by requirements made by individual healthcare professionals, insurers or providers, it may be the patient who is chosen.

Contesting patient choice

All of these models and policy programmes assume that patient choice is a benefit and a desirable attribute of healthcare systems for patients. But neither public nor private service users tend to conceive of healthcare provision as a conventional commodity subject to conventional consumerist exigencies (Baggott 2004). In a study of HIV clinics in England, Thorlby notes: 'Freedom to move (between) services had had an effect on the way that some of their services were designed. However, although most patients valued their right to choose, few had chosen to travel or change their hospital' (2006: ii). Further, there is evidence to suggest that patients are dependent on their GP's expertise to diagnose and select appropriate treatment and the overall quality of healthcare provision and value this over the ability to choose (Greener 2003). For many patients, particularly in countries with publicly funded national health services, an opportunity or requirement to identify and select their own doctors is both alien and alarming. While there is some evidence that patients would like increased access in terms of longer opening hours for general practice, there is far less evidence that they want to select healthcare providers. The implementation of choice policies can be disempowering and confusing for public services (Barnes and Prior 1995).

There is less consideration of the broader consequences the pursuit of the patient choice agenda has in terms of addressing health inequalities. People from deprived backgrounds are less likely to access general practitioner services, and when they do they are less likely to get referred for further investigation or treatment (Dixon *et al.* 2003). This suggests that the broad policy framework surrounding choice is under-developed since equity issues have not been considered. Appleby *et al.* point out that 'extending choice puts at risk a key objective of the NHS – equal access for equal need' (2003: 3), and argue that 'the benefits of extending choice are almost always at the expense of other benefits' (2003: 4). There are a multitude of reasons why people have differing resources to deploy to support their choosing. Limitations of access, social or educational capital, local availability of multiple provision all increase transaction costs and are unequally distributed across populations. As Björkman notes:

> But this model implies that demand, as expressed by purchasing power, should ultimately determine the supply and utilisation of healthcare services. It is thus, by definition, impossible for a perfect market to provide healthcare services according to need, regardless of ability to pay. Only if the groups with the greatest need for care would be those with the most resources for buying the care they need would the 'market forces' be a possible regulator of access to care.
>
> (Björkman 2004: 16)

Whilst patient choice within publicly funded healthcare systems creates an opportunity for people to choose various aspects of their healthcare (location, provider organisation, provider professional), this is often interpreted as a proxy for a willingness to pay for those services. Most systems with co-payments recognise that the consequences are likely to be regressive and only ameliorated through means-testing.

Cayton (2006) notes, that choice is essentially a function of exit, the ability to withdraw from a particular healthcare provider. However, since this depends on the ability to find a replacement, if this is not the case, choice may not exist. Here, the core policy issue of health inequalities emerges: since geographic location seems a reasonable indicator of health inequality (Chang *et al.* 2005), choice may not resolve this issue. Indeed greater choice may even add to a further health inequality burden. This is because those who are sick or elderly may not wish to, or be able to, travel; and the flight of middle-income 'choosers' may serve to exacerbate health inequalities for those left behind. This potentially problematic unintended consequence of the market system (involving selection, competition, success and failure) may also include enhanced hospital closures via the flight of those 'choosers' via the right of 'exit', resulting in further marginalisation of 'losers', who remain tied to their locality. Further, since significant elements of user groups of both healthcare and social care relate to disability and old age, it is likely that disenfranchised and 'hard-to-reach' groups may prove less able to enact choice, especially in context of geographic location of treatment.

Patient choice is promoted as a policy solution that drives competition between healthcare providers, whether they are organisations or individuals. 'The policy aims to improve access to healthcare by reducing waiting times for treatment, to promote a more responsive service and to introduce competition between providers' (Exworthy and Peckham 2006: 268). But in national systems such as the NHS or health services in Sweden and Finland, there is only limited scope for 'consumer choice' to influence and shape future provision. In such a system, centralised funding and target-setting mitigate the pressure that can be applied through individual choice.

A more overt explanation for the promotion of patient choice policies is pressure from the healthcare industry. This is because a prerequisite of choice is a plurality of providers, and this typically has been interpreted as a justification for creating market entry by private sector healthcare providers. For example, Pollock argues that the pursuit of particular policies may result in enhanced marketisation via 'the opening up of primary (and acute) care to new suppliers under the rubric of "patient choice" and "diversity"'(2004: 145).

The concept of choice has been based around a policy rhetoric of 'value added' and 'value for money'. The discourse immediately bifurcates to individual versus collective choice concerning issues such as hospital sitting, closure, reconfiguration, and service provision in the context of evidence-based health outcomes. Here, there exists the potential for conflict between individual and collective interests. This is because choice for some may limit and impact on the choice of others, since 'the pursuit of choice may put other healthcare objectives at risk' (Appleby *et al.* 2003: 32). Further complexities include the choice to not immunise children against mumps, which may have increased the risk to other members of the community to exposure. The operationalisation of choice therefore has the potential to interact or conflict with other values and aims embedded in a publicly funded health system such as equity, efficiency and quality.

> Choice is not a free good: its benefits must be weighed against its cost. It may also conflict with other desirable values in healthcare. Because of

the costs of creating choice, different individuals and different healthcare systems will have different views about the desirability of its benefits.

(Appleby *et al.* 2003: 35)

A central responsibility for publicly funded healthcare is to maximise the wellbeing of the population. As the WHO *Declaration on the Promotion of Patients' Rights in Europe* concludes, 'everyone has the right to such protection of health as is afforded by appropriate measures for disease prevention and healthcare, and to the opportunity to pursue his or her own highest attainable level of health' (WHO Regional Office Europe 1994: 1.6). However, policies promoting patient choice seem in conflict with those that promote collective involvement and maximum health gain of a population.

In order to maximise the collective benefit of healthcare and public health, planned healthcare delivery must be based on community and population need and experience. In this context, individual patient choice has the potential to undermine the opportunity of such planning, its implementation, and the scope for cost-containment (Rosenmöller, McKee and Baeten 2006). The influx of patients who are not planned for can be as challenging to a local health economy as the choice by members of the local community to seek and obtain healthcare services elsewhere. Such challenges become even more significant if planning at a local level must ensure sufficient excess capacity to allow the flexibility in provision that is the necessary precondition of patient choice.

Individual patients may attempt to circumnavigate problems with local services by choosing to receive treatment elsewhere, rather than engage in negotiation with those providers. Such an approach weakens the scope for collective action at a community level to address service inadequacies. Further, it detracts from the body of evidence about patient experience that can be used to evaluate and develop local services:

> Encouraging greater patient choice may actually undermine the influence of local democratic input into decision making, as patients choose to bypass local services rather than try to influence them through more collective means. The fundamental question here is how much value policy makers place on improving responsiveness of care compared with other objectives such as equity of access and efficiency.
>
> (Florin and Dixon 2004: 161)

The commitment to socialised medicine and a belief that health is fundamentally a public good with a distinct public value creates a special relationship between the state and society:

> The impact of markets on values and the precedence afforded to 'market' values over more 'social' values – efficiency, choice and quality rather than equity and planning and the ability of markets in health to support.
>
> (Dawson and Sausman 2005, in Slote Morris and Dawson 2006: 70)

There exists a potential dissonance between the collective 'greater good' ethos and practice of participatory engagement in healthcare provision and the more exclusive realms of individual choice concerning the location of treatment site. This is because, although private sector makes claims to co-provider enhanced healthcare provision, public services remain fundamentally a 'public good'. Further, since individual consumers tend to be driven by expectations, choice may raise those expectations to levels which healthcare may not have the necessary resources to meet.

Continuity of care is a significant test for individual patients who are encouraged to act as their own procurers and obtain healthcare from a range of different public, private and non-profit providers who are based locally, regionally and internationally.

> While some minor disorders can be managed as a single episode of care, many, especially where they involve an aggravation of a pre-existing condition, require communication with the individual's usual healthcare provider. The means that medical records must be accessible and understandable by different providers, there must be access to prescribed pharmaceuticals, and arrangements must be in place for follow-up assessments and rehabilitation.
>
> (Rosenmöller, McKee and Baeten 2006: 183)

If the range of providers includes private for-profit providers the sharing of information may be contested on the grounds of commercial sensitivity and ownership. Such situations are likely to lead to surplus treatment and testing as is apparent in the United States. More importantly the difficulties of creating a coherent framework for managing patients and providing continuity of care leads to an increasing fragmentation of services and undermines the integration of different types of treatment, care, and rehabilitation that will maximise recovery and the successful management of a condition.

One challenge to such a mix-and-match approach to provision encouraged by patient choice is the underlying culture of the nationally funded health service. Debate in the UK over the exclusion of some cancer patients from NHS services if they have previously sought private sector treatment highlights the tensions associated with seeking to implement an approach that is understood as undermining deeply held values within the culture of the NHS. As John Barron argued in the House of Commons:

> [T]he NHS does not allow co-payments, which involve a patient paying privately for a drug not funded by the NHS while continuing to receive the basic NHS package of care. If patients want to top up their care, Government policy requires that free NHS treatment be withdrawn. Often, treatment is eventually delivered within the NHS setting, but the patient is presented with the bill for all aspects of care.
>
> (Barran 2008: column 50WH)

The UK Government convened a review led by Professor Mike Richards the National Cancer Director of the consequences of additional private drugs for NHS care (Richards 2008). The issue emerged in relation to cancer treatments and the availability of drugs through the NHS, but has far broader consequences for the NHS: 'In reality, other health systems signal problems with this. Co-payments mean that – contrary to the founding principles of the NHS – access to treatment depends on ability to pay' (Finlay and Crisp 2008: a527). The consequences of cultural mismatch become even more apparent when the choice of service provider is abroad.

Within Europe, European Court of Justice rulings are reframing the opportunities for choice (Lowson *et al.* 2002; Exworthy and Peckham 2006), and there is some evidence that people are willing to travel abroad for treatment (Peckham 2004) but

> mobility of patients across Europe's borders is a somewhat marginal phenomenon as most patients prefer to be treated as near to home as possible, close to their relatives, in a system they are familiar with, and with providers who speak their language, where they know what they can ask for and what they can expect to receive.
>
> (Rosenmöller, McKee and Baeten 2006: 179)

Cross-border healthcare within Europe is currently not a significant threat to healthcare budgets or planning. As the European Commission notes, 'the current volume of patient mobility is relatively low, estimated at around 1 per cent of overall public expenditure on healthcare' (European Commission 2006b, citing 'Europe for Patients' Project, www.europe4patients.org).

Despite this low level of activity, the issue has prompted publication by the European Commission of a draft proposal for a *Directive of the European Parliament and of the Council on the application of patient's rights in cross-border healthcare* (European Commission 2008a). A previous draft of the Directive titled, 'Safe, high quality and efficient cross-border healthcare' was widely leaked over the last year and, although due to be published in December 2007, was eventually 'shelved at the last minute' (Mahony 2008). In relation to the patient choice agenda the current draft directive seeks to

> allow patients to seek any healthcare in another Member State that they would have been provided at home and reimbursed up to the amount that would have been paid had they obtained the treatment at home, but they bear the financial risk of any additional costs arising.
>
> (European Commission 2008a: 4–5)

The recent publication of new guidelines on medical tourism by the American Medical Association (AMA 2008) provides a clear indication of the broader global policy impetus behind this issue.

Operationalising patient choice

Models of patient choice are based on an implicit model of dyadic interaction: an individual patient choosing from a range of possible treatment options presented by an individual physician. Based on neo-classical economics, choice is framed by individual freedom, competition and user autonomy.

> To economists, choice is premised on the belief that the individual is all knowing, calculating, and an inherent utility maximiser, and thus the best judge of his/her own wellbeing, and that consumer sovereignty and giving people choice will force them to reveal their preferences.
>
> (Fotaki 2007: 1061)

These assumptions reflect neither the typical mode of treatment delivery, the physician's position, nor that of the patient – let alone the ways that decisions are arrived at.

When presented with a diagnosis a patient must spend time coming to terms with their situation, considering the implications of the diagnosis before being in a position to identify and evaluate responses in terms of potential courses of treatment. Decisions about treatment are often informed by media constructions of illness and broader understandings of health. The 'lay' understanding of illness is built from multiple sources only some of which may be deemed relevant by physicians. One way of illustrating the inappropriateness of the underlying assumptions associated with individual patient choice is to consider the situation of people who receive a diagnosis of cancer.

Studies of decision making by people diagnosed with cancer illustrate the active role that many patients pursue to understand the meaning of their diagnosis and identify potential strategies in response to their condition (Tritter 2008). Typically, people diagnosed with cancer seek a wide range of information either directly or with the help of family and friends (Leydon *et al.* 2000). The outcome of this 'research' is both a better understanding of their situation, and the basis to discuss and consider what treatment decision should be made. The process of decision making therefore takes time, energy, relies on multiple sources of information and discussion with various formal and informal social networks. Indeed in the first study of people's experience of cancer a key finding was that people wanted a speedy diagnosis, but then also a time to think prior to making a decision about treatment (Bell *et al.* 1996).

It is axiomatic that the vast majority of healthcare treatments are not delivered by individual physicians, but instead are the result of interdisciplinary teams of health professionals working in a range of clinical contexts. Nowhere is this complexity more apparent than in cancer care.

Cancer as a stigmatised and life-limiting illness may not be a typical case, but the ways in which people respond to their diagnosis and 'choose' a treatment does provide evidence of a lack of fit between the common assumptions underlying the ways in which patient choice is conceptualised. It also illustrates the ways in which patient choices are not individual but contingent and determined within a broad complex set of social networks and interactions. Physicians too rarely act alone and despite being potentially 'responsible' for treatment, medical interventions are the product of healthcare professionals working in interdisciplinary teams in a range of different clinical contexts.

Conclusion

The drive for greater choice in healthcare can be found in new public management arguments, whereby the market enthymemicaly[1] resolves the 'vices' of the public domain, such as inefficiency, bureaucracy and lack of accountability, with the pre-collectivist virtues of independence, self-reliance and privacy (see Hayek 1979). In this cosmology, those formally subject to the vagaries of unaccountable bureaucracy and professional paternalism of the medical model are transformed via the marketplace into active, self-realised healthcare customers. In this sense, problems of accountability and efficiency are translated and resolved through the introduction of choice. Based on the further evolution of healthcare consumerism, and the translation of patient into consumer, neo-liberal political economy emphasises exit, and displaces collective inter-relationships with market forces (Marquand 2004). The trend from a historic patient-centred model to a market-oriented one is being achieved via a linguistic turn which transforms the patient into a consumer. Here, the rhetoric of civil society is subsumed by one of individual choice; the shift in focus is apparent in the public record.

In this context 'choice' seems structurally associated with enhanced marketisation of healthcare provision. This is because, while the realm of the citizen is public, collective, and attentive to a rights-based ethos founded on notions of solidarity and consensus mediated by institutional regulation, the arena of the consumer is individual, autonomous, self-interested and based on the economic rationality of maximising personal benefits within market-based systems.

However, there are sets of core constraints on choice and since these constraints have not been sufficiently considered, this suggests that the broad policy framework surrounding choice is under-developed. For example, although patient choice via patient-focused care in the context of informed consent claims to equalise power differentials between health professionals and the community, the excess service capacity implicit in, and necessary for,

---

1 'Enthymemes take the form of an argument that comprises two propositions: an antecedent (A) and the consequent that is deduced from it (C); but where an implicit premise (P) is suppressed' (Morrell 2006: 379).

choice (since choice is essentially predicated on excess-capacity on stand-by) may tend to limit capacity for others to fulfil their healthcare needs. Further, the reframing of public responsibility as citizens for the health of the population to a patient's responsibility to identify and receive appropriate care has consequences for the relationship between citizen and the state and patient and healthcare professionals. As Henderson and Petersen suggest, 'The "good consumer" of healthcare is compelled to make choices, to exhibit appropriate "information-seeking" behaviour, and to behave in certain prescribed ways (consulting "relevant" expertise, taking the "right" medicine, engaging in personal risk management, and so on)' (2002: 3).

It bears repetition that the founding principles of the health systems in England, Sweden and Finland were comprehensiveness, universality and equity, in order to provide universal healthcare, based on need, free at the point of delivery, regardless of ability to pay. Consumerism undermines social solidarity – because it creates a mechanism for different individuals to compete for scarce resources against one another. The only way to make the value judgement about prioritising publicly funded health services for citizens is to involve them collectively in such decisions and create a basis for those with the greatest social and intellectual capital to demand their own care. These healthcare systems were designed around risk sharing, risk pooling and the promotion of collective values over individual choice.

4 Globalisation and global policy influences

Mapping the big picture

In this chapter we deal with two types of global influences on nation states. The first influence is the importance of globalisation on the financing, organisation and contents of health policies and the second is how global influences are mediated through international organisations or through policy exchange and learning between countries. There is a wealth of comparative analysis of healthcare reforms (see Chapter 2) in different countries (OECD 1992; OECD 1994; Saltman *et al.* 1997; Saltman *et al.* 1998; Freeman 1998; Docteur and Oxley 2003; Lister 2005; Oliver *et al.* 2005).

The focus of this chapter, however, is not on analysing the impacts of globalisation or of global agencies upon national health policy making or health systems, but rather exploring the actors and contexts in which globalisation and global policy influences take place upon i) healthcare reforms and in particular commercialisation of health services provision, and ii) public participation and citizen and patient rights. In other words rather than taking a country-based perspective we apply a global or transnational perspective on the actors, pathways and contents of policies as well as on the core assumptions, aims and emphases of these policies. Our focus is thus a deliberately global one and based on seeking commonalities and potential mechanisms of influence which could be relevant in explaining and moulding the nature and scope of health policies across England, Finland and Sweden.

The European Union is important both as an actor as well as a mediator of the impacts of globalisation. In addition to a 'domestic' influence within Europe (see Chapter 5), it increasingly seeks a role in shaping the external health policies of the European Union. The European Commission is already the main coordinator of external policies in the context of negotiations with international agencies in various sectors and thus has particular relevance to national policy actors and policy making.

Globalisation and global policies

The term globalisation is often used loosely or as another reference to global. We would like to separate these two concepts and emphasise globalisation predominantly as a process of economic integration and technological change, which is distinct from traditional international policies and policy actors or processes such as global climate change or global epidemics. We have excluded from our analysis the issues of global change and migration, although migration and minority group issues will be touched on in relation to the discussion on human rights.

The role and relevance of global policies can be addressed in relation to several policy spheres. In the areas we focus on, the global influence is mediated through:

1   the direct influence of global intergovernmental agencies in defining legally binding or non-binding guidance, standard-setting and evaluation. This includes the work of World Health Organisation (WHO) on health systems and services, the work of the OECD in the context of healthcare reforms and the follow-up and comparison of OECD countries and queues in healthcare. This also includes the work of the United Nations and health-specific aspects of human and social rights. In other words global and intergovernmental work with a *primary focus* on health;
2   the indirect influences of global intergovernmental agencies through other sectors, national policy change and commitments. This type of influence includes the role of trade agreements hosted by the World Trade Organisation, International Monetary Fund policies or the role of OECD in the context of regulatory and public management reforms. This includes activities such as those with human rights-related aims, which may have implications for health systems. That is, the main influence is mediated through *sectors other than health* based on activities with *other than health policy-related primary goals*. This is also the main source of global influence relevant to the globalisation process;
3   the direct and indirect influence of global nongovernmental organisations, corporations and campaigning. This includes campaigning directly in relation to national policies or indirectly in relation to regional or global policies. Consumers International, the work of International Association of Patient Organisations (IAPO) or the role of the International Federation of Pharmaceutical Manufacturers Associations (IFPMA) are examples of the type of actors wielding this type of influence;
4   the influence of *global ideas* on health channelled through other than governmental channels, such as epistemic networks, business and consulting community, learning and exchange. While global agencies act as intermediaries for ideas and changes, these are also transmitted outside global agencies. The promotion of Diagnostic Related Groups (DRGs), for example, has not been on the agenda of any particular international agency, but has been promoted through research, consulting and business communities due to the asserted benefits for creating markets and points of comparison (Lethbridge 2005).

The influence of globalisation overlaps with the role of global agencies and actors, but has to be considered in the context of expectations and impacts of globalisation on the scope and focus of national resources and in particular public sector funds. In terms of globalisation the indirect impact of international agencies and their work is often more important than their direct influence on health. Building and promoting global markets and structures that allow further development of service economies are usually set in the context of economic and commercial policy aims rather than as health policy priorities. Six main avenues for the impacts of globalisation can be identified:

1   the role and relevance of trade and investment agreements that are negotiated at bilateral, plurilateral and multilateral levels creating a broader legal framework for global economic integration (e.g. General Agreement on Trade in Services (GATS));

2   the role of international organisations in creating and promoting more market oriented structures and regulatory reforms (e.g. OECD work in relation to public services);

3   the impact of globalisation and active liberalisation of financial markets that creates vulnerability to economic crises and downturn (e.g. Finnish and Swedish economic downturn in early 1990s);

4   the influence of ideas and the expected consequences of globalisation on the provision of health (and public) services. This relates to how nation states try to cope with globalisation and what is considered and assumed possible and desirable;

5   the influence of global mobility, technological change and commercial opportunities on the organisation and nature of health systems. Globalisation also alters the context in which different options for health policies are elaborated. In particular this relates to issues of workforce and the nature of out-sourcing, contracts and continuity within the health sector;

6   the expectations about the opportunities that will emerge from globalisation and their impact on the health sector. This is reflected by increasing role of private investments, but by commercialisation as well. This entails measures which are guided by prospects for health sector commercialisation as an economic growth area for business and nation states.

International health policies and healthcare reforms

International agencies influence strongly the scope and nature of health policies and systems through suggesting and/or drafting policies and interventions at the global, regional and national levels. In the late 1970s and early 1980s the two major global health actors in health policies and especially healthcare policies were the World Health Organisation (WHO) and United Nations Children's Fund (UNICEF), which organised the Alma-Ata

Conference that led to the WHO's *Health for All* strategy (HfA) (WHO/ UNICEF 1978a). While the influence of these two organisations has perhaps been stronger in the developing world, the European regional office of the WHO developed its own *Health for All* strategies and targets and has provided an important forum of discussion and reflection for the European Ministries of Health (WHO Regional Office for Europe 1985).

The *Health for All* strategy and the *Declaration of Alma-Ata* formalised an emphasis on the role of the primary level healthcare. It also emphasised the role of other sectors and government's responsibility for the health of their citizens including responsibility for the provision of adequate health and social measures. The *Declaration of Alma-Ata* (WHO/UNICEF 1978b) recommended primary healthcare as a part of a comprehensive national health system and in coordination with other parts of the public sector. It stressed that people have the rights and duty to participate individually and collectively in the planning and implementation of their healthcare, stating that primary healthcare requires and promotes 'community and individual self-reliance and participation in the planning, organisation, operation and control of primary healthcare'.

The European Regional office of the WHO (WHO/Europe) prepared its own HfA strategy and targets (WHO Regional Office for Europe 1985). This emphasised the development of a healthcare system through effective community representation and that citizen participation in the planning and decision making about health is a fundamental principle (ibid.). While healthcare reforms as such were never part of the initial WHO agenda, aspects of the reform agenda were taken up by the WHO global work and in the 1990s in particular in WHO/Europe. However, while the WHO through the HfA had a clearly articulated position, its role in health services development and guidance has been more limited. This lower profile was partly due to the opposition by the United States to WHO engagement with health systems or health insurance in the early years, but also resulted from a lack of attention to the compiling of sufficient data and resources for global analysis. The lack of engagement by the WHO created the space and scope for the OECD to assume the leadership in terms of data gathering, analysis and comparisons across OECD countries.

In the late 1980s and early 1990s the OECD's comparative work focused on healthcare reforms and expanding documentation on the health data (OECD 1992; OECD 1994; Docteur and Oxley 2003). Both the OECD's public sector reform and its own Public Management Committee and Programme (PUMA) have influenced substantially the broader framework in which healthcare reforms were conceived and implemented. The World Bank engagement with healthcare reforms since the early 1990s has also contributed to the expansion of healthcare reforms in developing countries and countries in transition. At a global level and in relation to central and eastern European countries healthcare reforms became the main reference point for World Bank action. In the early 1990s the WHO/Europe took up this agenda through a set of studies on healthcare reforms that led to the Ljubljana Conference and resulting Charter (WHO Regional Office for Europe 1996).

The main message of the Ljubljana Conference was to frame healthcare reforms in terms of a set of health policy priorities and to limit the pressures for commercialisation. However, the WHO/Europe approach to healthcare reforms remained framed by new public management principles and an emphasis on government steering rather than rowing; nation states should organise rather than provide services.

In the late 1990s the global WHO policies incorporated much of the thinking emerging from the World Bank, most notably under the directorship of Gro Harlem Brundtland. This is most clearly apparent in the *World Health Report 2000* (WHO 2000), where an emphasis was put on government's role to steer rather than row and on promoting demand-based systems in which funding follows the patient. The approach that was promoted strengthened the link between performance and reward, and argued for increased plurality, competition and consumerism within health systems. The *World Health Report 2000* was a significant shift from an ideal of a needs-based healthcare delivery towards a demand-based one. In the new model citizen's participation was in many ways replaced by patient choice. It was also a shift towards private provision of health services, which were presented as more responsive to people's needs (Ollila and Koivusalo 2002).

However, at a global level, there has been a return to the original emphasis in the form of the *World Health Report 2008*, which focused on primary healthcare (WHO 2008a). Another contribution in the area has been the report of the Commission for Social Determinants of Health (WHO 2008b). The Commission had support from United Kingdom and Swedish governments, but it remains to be seen whether their recommendations, including the emphasis on universal health systems, will gain ground in practice.

The relationship between global policies and healthcare reforms in England, Sweden and Finland

The relationship between global policies and the given countries is based on a two-way process, where England can be seen as contributor to the global emphasis and agenda setting of healthcare reform policies as well as raising elements from the debates and discussions in the United States. This is reflected both in terms of epistemic networks and the choice of consultants hired by governments to develop healthcare reforms, but also in relation to the then conservative government policies and interest in reform strategies.

The role and relevance of thinking on healthcare reforms in the United States remains an important influence on health policies in England. This includes the development and implementation of internal or planned markets in health and the thinking of Enthoven (1993), which also directly and indirectly influenced reform policies in Sweden (Blomqvist 2004; 2007). The direct role of WHO on health policy making is less explicit; however, interview respondents in Finland and Sweden made reference to the WHO *World Health Report 2000*.

Since the 1990s the Finnish health sector has been reviewed twice by the OECD and OECD influence has also been conveyed by explicitly providing comparisons with other OECD countries, for example on waiting times. In this context the focus and basis of 'naming and shaming' through international comparisons seems to have shaped policy thinking and responses in all three countries. On the other hand, the OECD's influence is also mediated through other sectors and more general aspects of public sector reforms.

OECD and enhancement of the new public management agenda

Since the late 1970s an international trend that came to be called 'new public management' (NPM) has been influencing public sector policy reforms across both industrialised and non-industrialised countries. NPM has been understood to have arisen from two streams of ideas. The first stream emerges from the ideas of 'new institutional economics' that generated a set of administrative reform ideas built on a set of key concepts: contestability, user choice, transparency and incentive structures. The second stream draws on private-sector business models of *managerialism* and seeks to apply them to the public sector, in the tradition of the international scientific management movement (Hood 1991).

A key feature of NPM is the creation of a more market-oriented, private sector-type approach to the provision of public services (Mills *et al.* 2001). NPM can be seen as either a neo-liberal attempt to dismantle the welfare state and as a step towards a market-oriented service provision or as a way of improving the welfare state through increasingly efficient and better-quality services (Green-Pedersen 2002).

In the 1990s there was a wave of health sector reforms, and most countries, both industrialised and non-industrialised implemented reforms that had at least some of the following elements (Mills *et al.* 2001):

1   the restructuring of public sector organisations including decentralisation and bureaucratic commercialisation;
2   changing the way in which resources were allocated and paid to both organisations and individuals with the aim of strengthening the link between performance and reward;
3   the promotion of greater plurality and competition in the provision of healthcare services;
4   the increased financing of healthcare from non-tax revenue sources, such as user fees, social health insurance and private health insurance;
5   raising the role of the consumer in health system through enhancing the power and scope for consumer/patient choice and making health providers more accountable to community-based organisations.

While the advice of the WHO has been primarily concerned with health services, the World Bank and the OECD have advised and provided expert collaboration to support restructuring of the public sector as a whole including the health sector. For the industrialised countries the OECD has been instrumental in transmitting ideas about NPM, but it can be claimed it has been up to individual governments to decide how to deal with these.

The role of the OECD in public management dates from the end of 1980s. In 1990 the OECD founded the PUMA to support the improvement of the internal financial stability and enhance the effectiveness of public management across the OECD countries. PUMA emphasised serving individual countries. It became important in stimulating interest in the area of administrative reform among both OECD member governments and wider audiences and in formulating and propagating a particular mode of thinking about administrative reform (Premfors 1998).

In addition to PUMA and related work on public sector reforms and 'modernisation', the OECD has been important in promoting regulatory reform and trade in services. The OECD has also influenced European Union and European Commission activities in the area of internal markets and pressured for 'better regulation'. In the OECD's words from the website of the regulatory reform programme, it is aimed at: 'helping governments improve regulatory quality – that is, reforming regulations that raise unnecessary obstacles to competition, innovation and growth, while ensuring that regulations efficiently serve important social objectives' (OECD 1997).

The relevance of OECD influence at national level

The role of public sector and regulatory reform policies on countries is mediated through working groups, country guidance and guidance to the European Union. The OECD's report on regulatory reform for Sweden proposed that 'Sweden should instil more competition in the public sector, cut red tape and liberalise labour markets if it is to meet the challenge of an ageing population and maintain its high standards of social welfare' (OECD 2007).

In the context of OECD policies and public sector reform England remains a special case as, in many ways, it is at the leading edge of health policy reform. In terms of learning and policy diffusion it is also likely to have had more influence on Sweden and Finland than their policies have had on England. The role of OECD work in shaping of Finnish public sector policies, enhancing competition in public sector and contracting out services is rather clear and explicit in adoption of the agenda within the Finnish government. The OECD PUMA Committee is seen as an important forum where Finland has been an active participant (Lähdesmäki 2003).

The relevance of public management and OECD contacts must also be seen in the context of the respective power and the strength of sectoral administration. Engaging with Ministries responsible for finance, trade and industry or internal affairs has implications for the implementation of a health sector strategy. In many ways OECD advice can be seen as a mechanism for legitimating national policy priorities and change in other sectors. This process is apparent in Finland where the role of OECD work is seen to have enhanced and provided a neutral justification for national policies and priorities. However, the assessment for Sweden seems less clear and Carrol (2004) has argued that reforms have been primarily shaped by government policies and policy priorities.

Internationally many of the public sector management changes were introduced into national legislation in the 1990s and it is only now that their impact is becoming evident. The impacts and concerns relating to public sector and regulatory reforms within a nation state also need to be understood in the context of the regulatory framework that is developing within the European Union and in the context of global trade and investment agreements (see Chapter 5).

Trade and investment agreements and health services

The role of trade and investment agreements on health and public services was subject to direct and explicit public debate in the OECD negotiations on the Multilateral Agreement on Investment (MAI) in 1998 (OECD 1998). The OECD negotiations failed, but drew attention to processes that had taken place under the auspices of the World Trade Organisation (WTO).

Currently the main international negotiations relevant to health services relate to the General Agreement on Trade in Services (GATS) within the WTO and the negotiation of plurilateral and regional free trade agreements covering government procurement. The GATS covers trade in services and ultimately aims to liberalise all services. However, in contrast to the Agreement on Trade-Related Aspects of Intellectual Property Rights (TRIPS), governments have the possibility to choose which sectors and services to include in the agreement making them subject to its provision and also what kind of time-limited exceptions they would like to make. The GATS is important not only for market access by foreign providers to domestic markets for services, but also in relation to when, whether and how it affects the basis and scope of national regulatory policy space in particular within scheduled sectors bound by treaty provisions. While the GATS agreement aims to progressively cover more sectors, governments can decide what they want to commit to being covered by the Agreement during the negotiations.

The TRIPS was negotiated under the World Trade Organisation Uruguay round. In addition to patent protection the TRIPS covers copyrights, trademarks, geographical indications and technology transfer. The TRIPS incorporates flexible provisions so that governments can take into account some public health considerations; how and when these may be used is still unclear. However, the TRIPS is now complemented by additional and tighter bilateral agreements – the so called TRIPS + provisions – that exceed the requirements of the TRIPS and may limit the scope of these flexibilities.

The WHO guidance on services negotiations has emphasised prudence in terms of commitments and being explicitly clear what is committed (Fidler and Drager 2004). The WTO and World Bank associated expert guidance in the field of health has focused on the necessity of knowing what kind of commitments governments make (Adlung 2006; Luff 2003). The prospects of health tourism and problems of health insurance limitations to potential gains from liberalisation and out-sourcing of health services have also been raised for both developing and developed countries (Mattoo and Rathindran 2006; UNCTAD/WHO 1998).

Academic researchers and legal experts on international trade have drawn attention to the narrow GATS definition of public services and the likelihood that this would include services which are publicly financed but contracted out and provided by the private sector (Fidler 2003; Luff 2003; Krajewski 2003). This has particular relevance in relation to the current trend to enhance competition within public services and seeking forms of contracting out in the context of new public management. This clause would therefore not exclude health services if health services provision is contracted out to the private sector.

The expected benefits and problems of the GATS agreements relate to the ways in which it would tie national governments to complying with global governance arrangement based on commercial policy priorities. This so called 'lock-in' feature in terms of the liberalisation of services has drawn particular attention (Pollock and Price 2000; Grieshaber-Otto and Sinclair 2004; Mattoo and Wunsch 2004). While changing national commitments is possible, it requires compensatory measures elsewhere. For example, the United States had to change its commitments relating to online gambling as a result of a dispute settlement. It claimed it did not wish to bind online gambling and could not foresee this as part of the sports and recreational service sectors (Ortino 2006). While United States banned all internet gambling and treated foreign and national operators equally, the WTO dispute settlement, however, defined this as a zero quota for internet gambling setting a precedent that could restrict substantially regulatory policy space (Pauwelyn 2005; WTO 2005). As a result of this the United States initiated a process to withdraw this commitment from GATS.

The implications of GATS for national regulatory policy space are particularly in relation to the solidarity and universality of health systems. However, GATS does not limit the possibilities for governments to provide sufficient financing to cover the whole population. Despite this, it is likely that conflicts will emerge in term of cost-containment and the regulation of commercial service providers. It is also likely that it will have crucial implications on the ways in which cross-subsidisation can be undertaken as individualised financing options are more compatible with the free movement of services. While this has consequences for the redistributional aspects of health systems and thus to equity and solidarity, it is more likely that conflicts of interests will emerge in relation to the way governments subsidise and regulate health services.

Trade agreements and health services commercialisation

The relevance and importance of trade-related measures is based to a large extent on government decisions to include these services as part of trade agreements. In Finland and Sweden health services are not – at least not yet – included in the WTO schedules, whereas in the United Kingdom hospital services are already mostly scheduled (WTO 2009). However, even though the GATS agreement permits national regulation to achieve policy aims it must be compatible with GATS rules, as drafted in relation to universal service provision in the negotiation documents on domestic regulation (WTO 2008).

The role of national policy space is important as this relates to the ways in which governments can provide services through the market, subsidise service provision to ensure access in remote areas, cross-subsidise or limit patient choice or entry of providers to the given market. Issues that arise from the applications of GATS rules have similarities to those which emerge from the application of internal market rules on health services. However, in contrast to the current imposition of European Union internal market regulations on health services, governments have had a choice – or technically should have had a choice – on what they include in the agreements, whereas this has not been the case with respect to internal markets.

Considering the magnitude of regulatory measures in health services and the sensitivity of the sector, it has been emphasised that governments should know what they commit as they make commitments in the context of WTO negotiations in services. However, the changing nature of European Union governance has implied that, in contrast to national decision making, crucial negotiations are undertaken by the European Commission on behalf of Member States. The move towards more efficient trade policies implies a shift in European governance towards majority voting. However the proposed Constitutional Treaty would enhance this further. The implications of trade agreements upon national health systems are dependent on the ways in which they are financed and organised. This suggests that agreeing to a majority voting approach and not being able to fully influence the basis of commitments could be problematic and led to international agencies in the field of health advising against this proposal (Luff 2003; Fidler and Drager 2004; Adlung 2006).

The recognition of trade-related concerns and cooperation amongst the three countries was apparent during the negotiation of the proposed European Constitutional Treaty in 2004. All three countries cooperated in order to insert the health services clause in the European Union draft Constitutional Treaty which has been retained in the subsequent Lisbon Treaty (Treaty of Lisbon 2007). This clause is a watered down version of an earlier clause in the Nice Treaty, which defined the negotiation of trade in services in health, education and audiovisual services as a shared competence (Box 4.1).

Box 4.1. Treaty of Nice and Treaty of Lisbon provisions on commercial policy in relation to health services

Treaty of Nice, Article 133 paragraph 6:

6. An agreement may not be concluded by the Council if it includes provisions which would go beyond the Community's internal powers, in particular by leading to harmonisation of the laws or regulations of the Member States in an area for which this Treaty rules out such harmonisation.

In this regard, by way of derogation from the first subparagraph of paragraph 5, agreements relating to trade in cultural and audiovisual services, educational services, and social and human health services, shall fall within the shared competence of the Community and its Member States. Consequently, in addition to a Community decision taken in accordance with the relevant provisions of Article 300, the negotiation of such agreements shall require the common accord of the Member States. Agreements thus negotiated shall be concluded jointly by the Community and the Member States.

Treaty of Lisbon, Article 207 paragraph 4:

4. For the negotiation and conclusion of the agreements referred to in paragraph 3, the Council shall act by a qualified majority.

For the negotiation and conclusion of agreements in the fields of trade in services and the commercial aspects of intellectual property, as well as foreign direct investment, the Council shall act unanimously where such agreements include provisions for which unanimity is required for the adoption of internal rules.

The Council shall also act unanimously for the negotiation and conclusion of agreements:

a   in the field of trade in cultural and audiovisual services, where these agreements risk prejudicing the Union's cultural and linguistic diversity;
b   in the field of trade in social, education and health services, where these agreements risk seriously disturbing the national organisation of such services and prejudicing the responsibility of Member States to deliver them.

Treaty of Nice (2002) Consolidated version of the Treaty Establishing the European Community. Official Journal C 325. 24 December 2002.
Treaty of Lisbon (2007) Consolidated versions of the Treaty on European Union and the Treaty on the Functioning of European Union. Council of the European Union. 66/55/08 rev 1. Brussels 30 April 2008.

The role of state aid and government procurement stipulations may become more important in the context of global trade negotiations because of the European Commission's interest in enhancing negotiations on government procurement and liberalisation of services (European Commission 2006c). In this context trade agreements could become important for health policies, including the potential of out-sourcing of services to countries outside the European Union. Furthermore, the negotiations concerning Mode Four, which covers individuals travelling from one country to provide a service in another, is likely to become more important in GATS negotiations in future.

The challenge to national health policies is that the more governments engage with private sector actors in the provision of services and the greater the reliance on decentralisation of services, the more prone these are to being judged as being covered by trade agreements if governments have made commitments in these sectors. Further, the more plurality and contractual arrangements with providers the more government regulatory measures are required and the more educated they need to be in order to contract and oversee delivery appropriately (Saltman 2002). In Sweden and Finland legal measures to regulate healthcare have been limited if not barely present during the 1990s. These sectors have, however, been kept outside trade negotiations to maintain the possibility for government intervention. While foreign investment in these sectors has not been prohibited the governments have, at least so far, wanted to maintain a regulatory policy space within the sector so as to be able to act if necessary.

The importance of trade agreements, or internal market regulations, in both Sweden and Finland also comes from the potential to, knowingly or unknowingly, make commitments that limit the national policy space to regulate or subsidise in order to achieve particular health policy aims. In the context of trade negotiations one mechanism enhancing commitments has been the utilisation of so called 'stand still' arrangements in bilateral agreements. The 'stand still' arrangements bind sectors to an agreement on the basis of *existing legislation*. The lack of prohibitive legislation in relation to foreign investors or providers could then result in these sectors being considered *liberalised* and bound to the agreement. This was the case, for example, in relation to the Finnish negotiations of the EU–Mexico Free Trade Agreement with the initial inadvertent inclusion of health services as part of a general principle.

The attempt by governments to maintain areas of the public sector outside the remit of trade agreements can become problematic because of continued pressure of promoting markets and free trade. Rodrik (2007) has emphasised the implications and importance of policy space in contrast to merely focusing on market access in trade negotiations. This places particular emphasis on how trade negotiations are undertaken and the increasing role and competence of European Union in this process.

Health and social sectors as potential commercial export sectors

The incremental globalisation of health and social care has paralleled the expansion of commercial opportunities in other sectors. The commodification of health (Henderson and Petersen 2002) and health service provision implies a further phase of commercial development of the sector. Global markets and the prospects for out-sourcing and the opportunities provided by 'health tourism' have been seen as an avenue for developing countries to gather resources and for developed countries to save costs (UNCTAD/WHO 1998; Mattoo and Rathindran 2006). The globalisation of the health professional labour market is another aspect of commercialisation and particularly apparent in the UK's recruitment from commonwealth countries. The migration and mobility of health professionals in Europe is most prominent in relation to the United Kingdom, where this has been part of active recruitment policy with health professionals coming from outside Europe (Buchan 2006). The nature of cross-border mobility of professional workforce has become a more high profile global issue, particularly in terms of it consequences for limiting healthcare capacity in poor developing countries (Mensah 2005; WHO 2006).

The current impact of trade on health and social sectors is driven less by the unavoidable necessities of trade agreements than it is by the interests and focus of trade and industry representatives and finance ministries. This is reflected in specific measures in Finland and Sweden and particularly in the introduction of government procurement legislation that creates greater opportunities for private sector contracting out. In England the policy interests relating to trade and industry are more visible in the pharmaceutical and health technology sectors than in the context of commercial or export interests in relation to health services.

The role and relevance of trade policies in influencing national healthcare reforms and health policies echoes the pressures from the promotion of internal markets. While there are no trade disputes at the global level, the presence of contractual relationships and the development of a health services market is apparent in all three countries. It is likely that in addition to government trade and industrial policies further pressure will emerge from the interests of the service providers and pharmaceutical industries.

In both Sweden and Finland government agencies outside the Ministries of Health have also sought to develop health services as a commercial export sector. The provision of health services has become internationalised in the Nordic countries with Swedish H-Careholding now also own the Finnish private healthcare chain Mehilainen and is itself mostly owned by a British capital investment company and a Singapore government investment company (Carema 2008). In the United Kingdom the involvement of foreign companies in healthcare markets has been a central aspect of the contractual process with service contracts with South-African, Swedish and American operators.

The relevance of trade agreements is likely to become more important if there are disagreements over terms, operation of contracts, or if governments seek to return to their own public service provision. It is in this context that international agreements and their stipulations on state aid, monopolies in service provision and domestic regulation may become a concern. The intention of trade agreements has been to protect all providers from unfair treatment by governments. Where suppliers are large, however, they may have the litigation experience and capacity to use treaty provisions to promote their interests and rights to the detriment of an individual nation state or local government.

The influence of globalisation through demands on public sector budgets

The influence of globalisation on healthcare reforms in Finland and Sweden needs to be understood in the context of the economic crisis during the early 1990s and the consequences of this for public sector budgets and service provision. In both countries the economic crisis – in part due to globalisation and liberalisation of financial and capital markets – in the early 1990s resulted in greater government attention to productivity. In this context globalisation and an emphasis on limited public funds influenced the context in which health policies were framed and assessed. While the idea and provision of a 'welfare state' in both Finland and Sweden was supported in principle during the 1990s, it is clear that by the end of the decade the broader policy context of health service provision had changed substantially. Blomqvist (2004) has drawn particular attention to the ways in which the change in *how* services were provided has gained relatively little attention. Our interest is the extent to which international organisations and actors contributed to the design and choice of measures through which Sweden and Finland adapted to globalisation and the extent to which globalisation was applied in the context of national policy debates to enhance the commercialisation of health services.

In contrast to Finland and Sweden, the commercialisation of health services in England has taken place in a context of increasing rather than decreasing or stagnant resources. This is not surprising as, in Finland, municipalities which had earlier contracted out service returned to directly providing services after the economic crisis; in Finland scarce resources led to de-commercialisation (Koivusalo 2001). However, the process of commercialisation can be better explained through the shift of political power towards Ministries of Finance, Industry and Trade and their respective views of how to enhance the productivity and effectiveness of the public sector. As corporate lobbying and demand for change has been limited, explanations should be sought from the ways in which the Ministries of Trade and Industry and Finance operate. It is also in this context that the guidance and role of international actors and agencies becomes important. Organisations such as the International Monetary Fund convey their influence through personnel within Ministries of Finance, and in this way OECD and WTO policies and ideas gain ground in Competition Agencies or Ministries of Trade and Industry. The role of the OECD has also been important as a key reference group and actor seeking to *contextualise globalisation and shape responses* for public administration in key sectors.

Our assessment is that the role of OECD has been more explicit and influential in Finland than it has been in England or Sweden. This becomes more apparent in relation to policy reforms that aim to enhance competition and the contracting out of public services in the name of either productivity or cost-containment. This is most explicit in the national globalisation inquiry that took place during the Lipponen government (Valtioneuvosto 2004).

In England the national political context was different in the 1990s both in terms of policy pressures and resources. The commercialisation of the health sector under the first Labour government seems to have been most prominent in the areas where resources were available, including measures such as the Private Finance Initiative, contracting out services and creating independent bodies. The extent to which these measures were initiated on behalf of the Cabinet Office and Prime-Ministerial advisors rather than Department of Health highlights the political nature of the promotion of engagement with the private sector. However, the politics of healthcare reforms in the Nordic countries in the 1990s need to be set against the earlier efforts in England and the establishment of internal markets in healthcare. The policy direction in England is reflected in the OECD position promoting new public management reforms rather than the other way round (Armingeon and Beyeler 2004).

Citizens, consumers and public participation

The global influence on public participation and the role of citizens and consumers in healthcare has been at best limited. Healthcare has not been a major consumer issue, although this is changing in the context of more commercialised provision and more recently, in particular, with issues related to access to pharmaceuticals. However, global actors and influence in this area can be traced to five main pathways:

1   the role and relevance of United Nations stipulations on human and social rights
2   the focus on public participation in relation to *Health for All* and an emphasis on consumers and choice in the context of new public management and public sector reform
3   the role and relevance of international nongovernmental organisations, such as Consumer International, World Medical Association and the International Association of Patient Organisations in promoting consumer and patient rights and charters and participating in policy processes
4   in the context of commercialisation an emphasis on demand side puts greater attention to patient information, choice and the rights of citizens

5   the increasing relevance of lobbying and interest group policies that focus on 'stakeholder engagement' and 'public private partnerships' as key aspects of governance and accountability.

The extent to which these pathways shape national policies or have relevance in national debates is mediated by existing national policies and the distribution of political power. It is also clear that some of the processes relate more to rights and rights-based measures, whereas others focus more on participation and mechanisms promoting deliberative democracy and good governance.

United Nation treaties and global and regional commitments on human and social rights

Health and healthcare related rights are present in the United Nations Universal Declaration of Human Rights as well as the Convention on Economic and Social Rights which all three case study countries have signed. It is possible to separate stipulations that have a direct relevance to health and healthcare provision from those with indirect implications, for example in the context of discriminatory clauses, on how services are provided.

The two most directly applicable Articles are 21 and 25 (see Box 4.2) that focus on health and public services. However, after the Declaration was adopted by the international community in 1948, and the provisions moved to becoming legally binding commitments, a division between countries emerged. A western bloc argued that civil and political rights had priority while an eastern bloc supported social and cultural rights. This division resulted in, for example, the United States not being a member of the International Covenant of Economic, Social and Cultural Rights (ICESR). However, as 151 countries are current members of the Covenant it remains the most authoritative source for the articulation of rights to health: 'Article 12: Everyone has the right to the enjoyment of the highest attainable standard of physical and mental health' (UNHCR 1966).

The right to health, or the right to the highest attainable standard of health, was, however, first articulated in the WHO constitution in 1946. In international human rights law it is interpreted as a claim to a set of social arrangements – norms, institutions, laws, and an enabling environment – that can best secure the enjoyment of this right (WHO 2002).

Participation, the right to self-determination and taking part in public affairs, is also enshrined in the International Covenant on Civil and Political Rights (UNHCR 1966). This Covenant was created as a counterpart to the ICESCR. Participation was also integrated into the WHO *Health for All* strategy and focused on primary healthcare (Koivusalo and Ollila 1997).

The UN Human Rights Commission appoints a special rapporteur on the right to the highest attainable standard of health. Special rapporteurs undertake country reviews and the Review of Sweden highlights the discrepancy between the government's global policy endeavours and national policy

---

Box 4.2. Universal Declaration of Human Rights (United Nations 1948)

Article 21

1   Everyone has the right to take part in the government of his country, directly or through freely chosen representatives.
2   Everyone has the right of equal access to public service in his country.
3   The will of the people shall be the basis of the authority of government; this will shall be expressed in periodic and genuine elections which shall be by universal and equal suffrage and shall be held by secret vote or by equivalent free voting procedures.

Article 25

1   Everyone has the right to a standard of living adequate for the health and well-being of himself and of his family, including food, clothing, housing and medical care and necessary social services, and the right to security in the event of unemployment, sickness, disability, widowhood, old age or other lack of livelihood in circumstances beyond his control.
2   Motherhood and childhood are entitled to special care and assistance. All children, whether born in or out of wedlock, shall enjoy the same social protection.

United Nations (1948) General Assembly resolution 217 A (III) of 10 December 1948.

---

practices. Special Rapporteur Paul Hunt praised Swedish efforts, but pointed out problems in the context of national policies:

> Sweden is integrating human rights, including the right to health, into its *international* policies. At the international level, Sweden is committed to explicitly taking into account the right to health. Also, it encourages developing countries to explicitly take human rights, including the right to health, into account in their policy-making. In this respect, to its great credit, Sweden is among the world's leaders . . . But, strangely, the right to health is not yet explicitly and consistently integrated into Sweden's *domestic* policy-making. It is as though, when it comes to the right to health, Sweden does not practice at home what it preaches abroad.
>
> (Hunt 2007)

European regional focus on rights to health

The European Social Charter was established in 1961 and revised in 1996. The European Committee of Social Rights is the responsible body for monitoring compliance by states that are party to the Charter. The European Committee of Social Rights, like the European Court of Human Rights, is based at the Council of Europe in Strasbourg. The Council of Europe and the Commissioner for human rights report on the realisation of social rights; however, their power to exert influence on national policy decisions remains limited.

The right to health in the European Union is mediated through the Charter of Fundamental Rights of the European Union, which contains a number of provisions relevant to a right to health, although the charter does not include an explicit 'right to health' (Hervey 2006). However, in the context of health policies and healthcare reforms it does deal with healthcare, stating in Article 35 that:

> Everyone has the right of access to preventive healthcare and the right to benefit from medical treatment under the conditions established by national laws and practices. A high level of human health protection shall be ensured in the definition and implementation of all Union policies and activities.
>
> (European Charter 2000)

The role and relevance of the Charter is tied to its incorporation into the proposed EU Constitutional Treaties. According to Hervey, even without incorporation or other formal legal status the provisions of the Charter may influence health policy for a number of reasons. As an expression of the values that guide European Union as a polity, and in setting out interpretations of Community law and the obligations of the European Union institutions the Charter may prove an important influence (Hervey 2006).

The Council of Europe has engaged with patient rights and related concerns in adopting the recommendation that the patient be an active participant in their own treatment (Council of Europe 1980). In 1986 a recommendation was made on making medical care universally available (Council of Europe 1986).

In the early 1990s the WHO was actively involved in the promotion of patient rights in Europe. WHO/Europe prepared studies and surveys on the issue and published *The Rights of Patients in Europe* (Leenen *et al.* 1993) and drafted principles of patients' rights. In 1994 a European consultation was held in Amsterdam which adopted the principles of patients' rights and endorsed the *Amsterdam Declaration on the Promotion of Patients' Rights in Europe* (WHO 1994).

The difference between social and individual rights was central to these debates. What emerged was an understanding that while social rights are enjoyed collectively and cover aspects such as access to care and provision of adequate health services, individual rights in patient care are more readily expressed in absolute terms and can be made enforceable on behalf of individual patient. The rights of patients are defined in the WHO consultation.

Paragraphs 5.4–5.6 of the Consultation report incorporate aspects of human rights and values in healthcare, rights related to information, consent, confidentiality and privacy, care and treatment, where choice seen in the context of a broader set of rights and obligations:

> 5.4. Patients have the right to continuity of care, including cooperation between all healthcare providers and/or establishments which may be involved in their diagnosis, treatment and care.
>
> 5.5. In circumstances where a choice must be made by providers between potential patients for a particular treatment which is in limited supply, all such patients are entitled to a fair selection procedure for that treatment. That choice must be based on medical criteria and made without discrimination.
>
> 5.6. Patients have the right to choose and change their own physician or other healthcare provider and healthcare establishment, provided that it is compatible with the functioning of the healthcare system.
>
> (WHO Regional Office for Europe 1994)

In contrast to the earlier emphasis by the WHO on patient rights, the role of choice is much more prominent in the WHO Ljubljana Charter (WHO Regional Office for Europe 1996). Section 6.2 of the Charter emphasises the contribution of citizens' voices and choices in shaping healthcare services:

> 6.2 Listen to the citizen's voice and choice
>
> 6.2.1 The citizen's voice and choice should make as significant a contribution to shaping healthcare services as the decisions taken at other levels of economic, managerial and professional decision-making.
>
> 6.2.2 The citizen's voice should be heard on issues such as the content of healthcare, contracting, quality of services in the provider/patient relationship, the management of waiting lists and the handling of complaints.
>
> 6.2.3 The exercise of choice and of other patients' rights, requires extensive, accurate and timely information and education. This entails access to publicly verified information on health services' performance.
>
> (WHO Regional Office for Europe 1996)

While earlier European consultations focused on comprehensive patient rights, the WHO Ljubljana Charter sets them clearly in the context of choice and the implications of this for the provision of health services. The relationship and critical assessment of the priorities of healthcare reforms was more explicit in the fifth conference of Health Ministers on *Equity and patients rights in the context of healthcare reforms* in Poland in 1996 (Council of Europe 1997). The final text emphasised the need to take better account of equitable access and citizens' and patients' participation. The relationship to the reform process as well as the absence of users' or citizens' role in the process was clear in the articulation of the 'current concerns':

- the predominance of budgetary constraints at national level in many countries, leading to serious cuts in health expenditure despite the relative priority of healthcare as compared with other social goods, thus counteracting the necessary development and implementation of a sound public health policy;
- withdrawal of state and collective responsibility for health promoting environments, health and social security, leaving too much to market forces and allowing for a growing health divide, in particular between employees and those who are not part of the work force;
- in some countries the tendency towards an increasingly influential role for budgetary authorities (Ministries of Finance) leading to a vanishing leadership role for the Ministries of Health, which can sometimes contribute to their divided loyalty between the public and the governments;
- a change in the respective roles, responsibilities and entitlements between patients, providers and payers, the latter playing a dominant role;
- the fragmentation and relative weakness of the users' voice lacking institutional possibilities to put health on the political agenda, to mobilise the public or to attract the attention of the media.

(Council of Europe 1996)

While the process of healthcare reforms slowed during the late 1990s, the Council of Europe's work on patient rights resulted in an official recommendation with five additional core recommendations. Further explanatory guidelines (Council of Europe 2000) were framed in terms of citizen and patient participation in the democratic process and in creating legal structures and policies that promoted this. The recommendations also encouraged the growth of healthcare user organisations. In this context the guideline promoted a deliberative approach to decisions about health systems, not merely in respect to individual patient care.

The role of international nongovernmental actors on policy options

The role of human rights organisations and advocacy is prominent in the context of global policies dealing with issues with discriminatory potential and practice. However, while recognising the breadth and importance of different rights-based policy issues and agendas, including those associated with reproductive rights, disability, minority groups, gender or access to medicines, we focus on rights to healthcare and patient rights, covering the role of international consumer organisations, international professional organisations, international patient organisations and international industry related-groups or astro-turf[2] groups.

For example, Consumer International works primarily through consumer mobilisation and focuses on pharmaceuticals and the marketing of pharmaceuticals internationally. The role of their international focus is likely to be smaller than in relation to national policy developments in health services. In consumer-related matters the relevance of international organisations and their activities seems much stronger in relation to pharmaceuticals and pharmaceutical policies (see Chapter 5). The international context of consumer politics in European countries remains primarily related to EU policies.

In terms of international influence the role of medical professional associations and trade unions is important in bringing issues into the policy agenda, but has had limited impact. The World Medical Association (WMA) *Association Declaration on the Rights of the Patient* was adopted initially in 1981, revised in 1995 and further edited in 2005 (WMA 2005). However, it is likely that the importance of the WMA as an actor is primarily in the broader development of international and regional legal guidance, rather than as a direct influence on particular national policies. This is reflected in the fact that there are few references to the Declaration that emerged in our documentary analysis or interviews with professional associations.

The impact of patient organisations and their international affiliations on policies that focus on social or patient rights has also been limited. However, the International Association of Patient Organisation's *Declaration on patient-centred healthcare* expresses five principles: respect, choice and empowerment, patient involvement in health policy, access and support and information (IAPO 2006). Thus, while IAPO has a specific statement on patient involvement (IAPO 2005) it has produced no statement related to social or patient rights.

The role of international patient associations seems to be primarily campaigning on specific international issues with a focus on the global or international context (e.g. the Diabetes Resolution in the United Nations). In terms of global influence and the influence of globalisation, think tanks and representatives of industry need to be considered. It is clear that in the Finnish and Swedish context national think tanks representing, or with close ties to, business and industry interests or employers associations have been influential in promoting the need for healthcare reform and competition at a national level (see Chapters 7 and 8). One example operating at the European level is Consumer Powerhouse, which takes an active part in health policy debates, but is far more associated with industry than consumer interests.

---

2 Astro-turf groups have been discussed in the context of public relations strategies with respect to various issues with cases reported as well in relation to health (see e.g. Lyon and Maxwell 2004; O'Harrow 2000).

Another example of pan-European influence is the Stockholm Network, which has an office in London and articulates a pro-consumer choice position in healthcare.

The demand for new treatments and medical products is vital to the pharmaceutical industry. It is in this context that the promotion of patient choice, information, training and public–private partnerships can be seen as part of a broader commercial endeavour. It is also in this context that pharmaceutical industry support and promotion of patient rights and participation should be understood.

Conclusion

The influence of global agendas on healthcare reforms and on citizen's rights can be seen to flow through the 'economic' focus of the World Bank, OECD and related institutional actors (see e.g. Koivusalo and Ollila 1997; Lister 2005). Patient and citizen rights in contrast are more likely to be raised through the 'rights' channels that focus on law and legislative changes. These two influences tend to take different routes and are not necessarily easily reconciled.

International trade agreements provide a third route by creating a legal framework that influences how and on what basis governments can regulate, subsidise and organise the provision of health services. The promotion and expansion of healthcare reforms incorporating market mechanisms such as the purchaser–provider split and the increasing role of private sector providers relying on government 'steering not rowing' has given these legal frameworks greater traction in health systems.

While citizen and patient rights have been promoted through global and regional human and social rights commitments and their implementation, healthcare reforms are part of the broader agenda of global public sector management and regulatory reform. The relevance of global trade policies in influencing public sector and health reforms has been limited within the European Union; however, it is clear that the role of trade agreements needs to be seen in terms of promoting changes that create opportunities for multinational interests and that this influence is likely to grow in the future.

The importance of patient and citizen rights has, with the exception of the promotion of patient choice, been predominantly a matter of global and regional human and social rights related commitments. The focus on public participation and deliberative democracy is also apparent, particularly in Council of Europe recommendations. The relative unimportance of patient choice as part of the more 'rights-based' global agenda contrasts with its strong presence in both national and European policy debates.

5   The European Union
Trading in healthcare or building a healthier Europe?

The role and relevance of the European Union to health systems and their functioning has changed over the last ten years. When the European Union was established its relevance was not generally anticipated, and indeed even when Finland and Sweden joined the European Union it was with public and policy assumptions that the European Union would have little impact on health and social services. The subsidiarity principle that governs European Union functions was understood to ensure that decision making in these fields would be done on the basis of national policy priorities with no European Union influence. While the concerns of the Nordic countries over joining the European Union were more related to the worries over its impact on welfare states, the situation for the United Kingdom was different. The United Kingdom was one of the founding members of the European steel community and a participant in the Rome Treaty at the beginning of the integration process. The problem for the United Kingdom was not that Europe would affect the welfare state but, particularly apparent during the Thatcher era, that new European social regulations would be imposed on the United Kingdom. Europe was considered too social and insufficiently free-market oriented and this is still reflected in some United Kingdom positions concerning the European Union.

In this chapter we begin by discussing and addressing the changing legal context and the understanding between the European Union and Member States in general, and in particular relation to health. We then discuss three different elements that have more direct relevance to healthcare, markets and public involvement. We start by exploring the expanding role of the European Union in the field of health services. Second, we analyse the ways in which decisions outside the health sector influence national policies within the sector. Finally, we seek to understand the role of citizen involvement, trust and public participation in the European Union and in health policies in particular.

The constitutionalisation of the legal framework of the European Union

At the end of the day the role and relevance of the European Union is defined in the context of the treaties from which it gains its legitimacy. The importance of the legal treaties is of course set in the context in which these are interpreted and utilised. The EU and EC treaties guarantee four fundamental market freedoms: free movement of goods, services, people and capital. These form the basis of the single market framework and include freedom of establishment as well (Article 43 in TEC or Article 49 in the Treaty of Lisbon; see also Box 5.1). The four freedoms form a crucial part of the European Union substantive law (see Barnard 2007).

Box 5.1. Treaty of Nice and Treaty of Lisbon provisions on public health and health services

Treaty of Nice, Article 152 paragraph 5:

5. Community action in the field of public health shall fully respect the responsibilities of the Member States for the organisation and delivery of health services and medical care. In particular, measures referred to in paragraph 4(a) shall not affect national provisions on the donation or medical use of organs and blood.

Treaty of Lisbon, Article 168 paragraphs 2 and 7:

2. The Union shall encourage cooperation between the Member States in the areas referred to in this Article and, if necessary, lend support to their action. It shall in particular encourage cooperation between the Member States to improve the complementarity of their health services in cross-border areas.

    Member States shall, in liaison with the Commission, coordinate among themselves their policies and programmes in the areas referred to in paragraph 1. The Commission may, in close contact with the Member States, take any useful initiative to promote such coordination, in particular initiatives aiming at the establishment of guidelines and indicators, the organisation of exchange of best practice, and the preparation of the necessary elements for periodic monitoring and evaluation. The European Parliament shall be kept fully informed.

7. Union action shall respect the responsibilities of the Member States for the definition of their health policy and for the organisation and delivery of health services and medical care. The responsibilities of the Member States shall include the management of health services and medical care and the allocation of the resources assigned to them. The measures referred to in paragraph 4(a) shall not affect national provisions on the donation or medical use of organs and blood.

Treaty of Nice (2002) Consolidated version of the Treaty Establishing the European Community. Official Journal C 325. 24 December 2002.
Treaty of Lisbon (2007) Consolidated versions of the Treaty on European Union and the Treaty on the Functioning of European Union. Council of the European Union. 66/55/08 rev 1. Brussels 30 April 2008.

The questions on health and the European Union have been framed in terms of subsidiarity and competence; decisions which are best taken at national level should not be taken at a European level. However, in the context of European Court of Justice decisions, interpreting the four freedoms, giving a stronger emphasis on internal market principles and industrial policies between countries, implies a change in how subsidiarity and competence are interpreted in relation to health and social services.

Social policy and health policy studies based on comparative approaches have traditionally emphasised the lack of convergence either in terms of financing or organisation of care as no particular organisational form for national health system has become dominant. On the other hand, focusing on convergence may undermine the ways in which commercialisation has influenced national health systems in different ways depending on how these are financed and organised. In other words, the issue is whether health systems have all moved towards a particular direction within their broader organisational structures (see Evans 2005).

While the basic freedoms were agreed decades ago, the importance of these and the constitutionalisation of the role of the European Union has become relevant to national policy and decision making only lately. The emphasis on the importance of the legal context was first argued in the context of neo-functionalism with a prediction that influence of the European Union would expand to other fields (Haas 1958). This basic assumption has also been emphasised to explain the changing context of the European Union and its relevance to health policies.

While the broader establishment of internal markets was set in force in the Maastricht Treaty, this became more evident only later in the 1990s. For example, when Sweden and Finland joined the European Community it was still argued strongly that the European Union had nothing to do with social and health services, which were of national competence. Furthermore, the direction was more towards strengthening of particular policy aims through the European Union. In the Amsterdam Treaty, the exclusion of health services was explicit and clear in terms of competence, with a strong emphasis on subsidiarity in relation to public health (Article 152). It could even be argued that had Finland and Sweden at the time of joining to the European Union known that this would result in the acceptance of internal markets as the guiding principle for health service organisation and regulation, the results of the vote to join to the European Union might have been different.

In the early 1990s the role of the European Union in health and social policies was predominantly considered as a potential field for cooperation and strengthening of the 'Social Europe'. This emphasis was and has been particularly evident in England which, before the New Labour reign, was not willing to participate, and where the European Union was seen as more progressive in terms of social policies. The European Union would bring new employment regulations and other social regulations not currently on their agenda. This emphasis has gained ground in the context of the so-called soft or political influence of the European Union in the field of employment policies and leads also to the expansion of European role in the field of social policies and social policy making. This does not mean it could not affect health policies in practice. One example is the Working Time Directive, which has had broad implications to health systems and has been in England perhaps the most commonly brought up reference point when discussing impacts of the European Union upon national policy options and choices. Social policy aims are also reflected in the Treaty of Nice (2001). While England and the United Kingdom remain cautious in terms of the European Union, particularly in relation to employment policies, the direction of the European Union influence is markedly different in health services.

In the late 1990s the role of legal and constitutional elements of the European Union became articulated more prominently. While the European Court of Justice had made decisions on health-related matters prior to the Kohl and Decker cases, the political context and argumentation on health-related matters had changed in Europe. The first Treaty-driven process has been followed by a second, more political and legislative process utilising European Court of Justice decisions and interpretations. The European Court of Justice cases thus became the basis for the articulation of three processes that could be articulated: first, the inclusion of health services in the context of broader internal markets and thus under internal market regulations; second, the opening of scope for political integration in the context of the open method of coordination so as to ensure government compliance with internal market regulations; and third, the broadening of the mandate of the European Union competence beyond public health to cover health services as well.

The general emphasis in the European Union has now shifted towards an emphasis on the four freedoms, internal markets and the enhancement of the European Union role in the field of trade and external policies. These aims have sought to be secured and strengthened on the basis of amendments to treaties and the new Constitutional Treaty. The political emphasis of this was articulated in the context of the Lisbon Strategy, which had its emphasis in enhancing competitiveness of the European Union. The European Court of Justice decisions as well as the European Commission interpretation and use of these decisions were of importance in the context of the service directive communication (European Commission 2004a), where health and social services were actively included.

The first draft of the Constitutional Treaty and several elements in the initial negotiations sought to expand the competences of the European Commission, and its focus on health, beyond public health. This is also reflected in the text of the proposed Lisbon Treaty (Article 168 paragraph 7), which rephrases the long-standing Article 152 limiting competence to public health, 'Community action in the field of public health shall fully respect the responsibilities of the Member States for the organisation and delivery of health services and medical care' (Treaty of Nice 2002). The Treaty process has also enhanced European Union competence in relation to trade policies with a shift from shared competence on health and social services in the Treaty of Nice to a strongly conditional 'emergency break' measure in the proposed Constitutional Treaty and its later revisions (see Box 4.1)

While the process of establishing a Constitutional Treaty for Europe has been hampered by citizen votes, it is likely that constitutionalisation is part of the future processes within the European Union. However, the scope for social rights in the Constitutional Treaty is dependent in part on the standing and recognition of the EU Charter of Fundamental Rights within the Treaty (see Fredman 2006; Hervey and Kenner 2006). However, in England, consideration of the EU Charter of Fundamental Rights is further affected by the opt-out by the United Kingdom.

It is important to note that there were initial joint activities between Member States to exclude health services from internal markets, and thus clarify the relationship between internal markets and healthcare, even though these efforts failed to produce a result in the overall negotiations. The United Kingdom, Finland and Sweden, for example, were all involved in articulating this position, but the issue did not gain sufficient priority in the overall negotiation process. However, it does reinforce the potential to seek an exception for health and health services.

Should these efforts have been realised they would have clarified the relationship between healthcare and internal markets, leaving European cooperation on health to Ministries of Health and expanding the role of the Directorate-General for Health and Consumers (DG Sanco) on the basis of health policy priorities.

The challenge of the current processes and emerging legitimisation of European Union action can be seen in the light of the Commission draft directive on patient rights in cross-border healthcare in July 2008 (European Commission 2008a). The aim of this proposal is to address uncertainty in cross-border healthcare; however, in light of its contents it is likely to increase rather than decrease uncertainty about patient rights in cross-border healthcare. The proposal is based on Article 95 of the Treaty, which has its focus on the functioning of internal markets. The draft directive also twists the orig-inal intentions of the European Council statement on common values (Council of the European Union 2006). This statement was critical to the application of internal market principles to health systems, and which invites the European Commission to ensure that common values and principles contained in the statement are respected when drafting specific proposals concerning health services. However, the Commission proposed draft directive uses this statement to legitimate its action in expanding the Commission's competence in health services and taking health services within internal market priorities, while using the common values as basis for harmonisation and level and practice of reimbursement to be agreed.

The draft directive on patient rights in cross-border healthcare, not only lacks clarity with respect to the rights of patients, but also, obscures the location of competence in decision making on regulatory aspects of health services provision. However, even if it does not become a directive, it draws attention to particular issues with respect to the nature of the process of defining competence in regulating health services in Europe. This process not only relates to the issue of free mobility or equal treatment for patients from different Member States as a matter of consumer rights, but also further legitimates and strengthens the case where competence on health services resides and how this could affect the organisation and financing of health within Member States, more broadly. Member States appear to be focused on the relatively small magnitude of the actual cross-border movement or in pursuing efforts to maintain their scope for pre-authorisation. In doing so they may fail to adequately consider the extent to which the process has broader significance for the future. The draft directive provides evidence of the potential to limit the scope of national governments and national policy space to undertake unilateral cost-containment measures, pursue cross-subsidisation agendas and maintain oversight within health systems. Such actions are potentially threatened if the European Commission considers such activities as limiting the functioning of internal markets more than is necessary or proportional to the desired impact.

The European Union and health services

European Court of Justice decisions are claimed to form the basis for the shifts in the European Union role in health services. Since the first decisions with respect to the so-called Kohl and Decker cases in 1990s there have been several further cases on the matter (ECJ 1998a; ECJ 1998b; ECJ 2000). It was initially perceived that internal market rules would be more problematic in the context of social insurance institutions, however the Watts case fundamentally changed this perception (ECJ 2006). The Watts case applied directly to the United Kingdom and it was no longer possible to claim that internal market rules would not apply also to NHS type of services.

As a result, the European Court of Justice decisions served as grounds for a high-level group on internal markets and health services in 2001 (High Level Committee 2001), which concluded that health services are within the internal markets and thus subject to related law. As the Commission derives its legitimacy of action in particular from internal markets rules and regulations, the expansion of the health mandate was done through two processes: first, the initiation of open method of cooperation on the matter, and second, through Commission communications and initiatives. This was further complicated by the fact that activities were divided between DG Employment, Social Affairs and Equal Opportunities, which was accountable for an open method of coordination and dealt with services of general interest issues, and the DG Sanco, which prepared a draft directive on cross-border health-care. These competing efforts were challenged – if not run over – by the DG Enterprise inclusion of health services in the services directive. As part of the debate and discussion on health service directive, health services were carved out from the services directive and the task of sectoral directive was shifted to the health DG, DG Sanco.

In 2006 the Commission launched a consultation on the role of European Commission with respect to health services (European Commission 2006b). The nature of this consultation made it clear that it was an issue of how, rather than whether, the scope of action should be enhanced. While it was recognised that cross-border trade covers only an estimated 1–2 per cent of total healthcare costs, it was still argued why this had to be addressed by the European Commission. The consultation was run alongside another on Health Strategy, which set the context of the expansion of the Commission mandate to health services. While cross-border issues have been traditionally dealt with in the context of social security coordination, the emphasis on cross-border mobility and access to information on healthcare in other Member States has clearly been on the Commission agenda within DG Sanco. The Commission's communication and directive proposal on cross-border healthcare was leaked in autumn 2007, but was shelved until summer 2008, when the final document emerged under the title of patient rights.

The high-level group work has supported this process in 2004–2006 through the production of working documents and materials and in suggest-ing a broader role in the field of health services for the Commission. On the other hand, in the DG Employment the process of an open method of coor-dination (OMC) has continued and has provided a basis for activities. The responsibilities and nature of the process reflected in the statement related to the future tasks for the OMC seem to be, however, more in adjusting national strategies to fit the Treaty of the European Union rules than in sup-porting national strategies as envisaged in the title of the Communication *Modernising social protection for the development of high-quality, accessible and sustainable healthcare and long-term care: support for the national strategies using open method of coordination*. It is clearly indicated as part of this that:

> Responsibility for the organisation and funding of the healthcare and elderly care sector rests primarily with the Member States, which are bound, when exercising this responsibility, to respect the freedoms defined and the rules laid down in the Treaty. The added value of the 'open method of coordination' is therefore in the identification of chal-lenges common to all and in support for the Member States' reforms.
>
> (European Commission 2004b: 11)

In health and social services another focus governed by the DG Employment has been set in the context of services of general interest. In the discussion on services of general interest particular attention needs to be put on the one hand to the definition of services of general interests, which are not subject to internal market regulations, and on the other hand to services of general economic interests, which are subject to internal market regulations. The way in which the latter group has been defined, implies that services of general interest will remain a residual category of services, which are not contracted out or put on the markets, in other words defined more as services which are of no economic interest. This definition is discussed already in the Green Paper dividing services of general interest in three categories of which two are services of economic interest covered by internal market, competition and State aid rules, and a third, which deals with non-economic services:

> Services of general interest of a non-economic nature and services without effect on trade between Member States are not subject to specific Community rules, nor are they covered by the internal market, competition and State aid rule of the Treaty. However, they are covered by those Community rules that also apply to non-economic activities and to activities that have no effect on intra-Community trade, such as the basic principle of non-discrimination.
>
> (European Commission 2003: 11)

This approach is further recognised in the White Paper, which is now geared more towards addressing user views, but emphasises that it is a matter of *political choice* of governments to provide services through markets, rather than through directly tax-funded measures:

> While in principle the definition of the missions and objectives of social and health services is a competence of the Member States, Community rules may have an impact on the instruments for their delivery and financing. A clear definition of the distinction between the missions and the instruments should help to create more clarity with a view to the modernisation of these services in a context of evolving user needs while preserving their specific nature in terms of the particular requirements of, amongst others, solidarity, voluntary service and the inclusion of vulnerable groups of people. Clarifying this distinction will in particular help Member States which use market-based systems to deliver social and health services to anticipate the possible impact of EU competition law on them. It will of course remain a matter of political choice for Member States whether to use such systems or to provide services directly via tax funded State agencies.
>
> (European Commission 2004c: 16–17)

The issue of services of general interest consequently became a broader concern of variety of actors. This resulted in actions and new measures emphasising user rights, equity and universal service provision, which were included as part of the proposed Lisbon Treaty added protocol, in order to respond to the concerns that resulted in the unsuccessful popular vote. However, the emphasis in Article 2 of the protocol of Member State competence in the Treaty protocol covers only non-economic services, which were already defined as a residual category of services of no trade interests (Treaty of Lisbon 2007) (see Box 5.2).

Box 5.2. Protocol 26 on services of general interest Article 1 and 2

Article 1

The shared values of the Union in respect of services of general economic interest within the meaning of Article 14 of the Treaty on the Functioning of the European Union include in particular:

- the essential role and the wide discretion of national, regional and local authorities in providing, commissioning and organising services of general economic interest as closely as possible to the needs of the users;
- the diversity between various services of general economic interest and the differences in the needs and preferences of users that may result from different geographical, social or cultural situations;
- a high level of quality, safety and affordability, equal treatment and the promotion of universal access and of user rights.

Article 2

The provisions of the Treaties do not affect in any way the competence of Member States to provide, commission and organise non-economic services of general interest.

Treaty of Lisbon (2007). Consolidated versions of the Treaty on European Union and the Treaty on the Functioning of European Union. Council of the European Union. 66/55/08 rev 1. Brussels 30 April 2008.

While DG Sanco and DG Employment seem to make competitive openings in the field of health, their actions seem to follow to a large extent internal markets rules and regulatory needs. Thus, rather than balancing health and social protection needs and internal market regulatory measures, these seem to bring in the internal market requirements as the core building block for work. The question that needs to be asked is to what extent their core role is increasingly becoming understood as bringing health and social sectors into compliance with internal market and as means of increasing economic competitiveness in the context of the Lisbon Strategy.

On the other hand, more Member State led processes in the Council have been able to formulate a statement on common values that emphasises solidarity and equity (Council of the European Union 2006). However, in the health strategy White Paper it is argued that these values should be expanded and citizens' empowerment should become a core value as healthcare is becoming increasingly patient centred and individualised. Further, it argues that the Commission needs to build on the work of the citizens' agenda and take citizen's and patient's rights as a key starting point in health policy (European Commission 2007a).

Member States appear to engage continuously as part of Council work to highlight health issues and needs and how these are not necessarily in line with internal market focus. The challenge in this area is that the Commission seems to be able to operate only in the context of internal markets and considers its main task to ensure Member States make adjustments to follow requirements of internal markets. While the Commission appears to be willing to act on behalf of patient and citizen rights, its actions have taken place in the context of internal markets. This is the case, for example, with respect to the fate of the patient rights in cross-border healthcare directive, which gives little support to these rights in the broader framework in which health systems function.

Internal markets, trade, employment and industrial policies

As the free movement of people, services, capital and goods has been reinforced by European Court of Justice decisions and interpretations, this has led to repercussions within European Community politics. While it is recognised that governments may depart from requirements set on the basis of financial sustainability of health systems, it is unclear how much is enough to legitimise the use of this claim. In other words it is not clear what kind of arguments could be approved to be legitimate in this context. This is of importance for health systems, but also in relation to other measures, such as issues related to state subsidies, government procurement and public services.

While European government procurement directive allows exclusion of health services as services not included in the directive, there is an emerging process also in this field on the basis of recent ECJ court interpretation, which has in practice argued that on the basis of the four freedoms, procurement measures below the threshold level and across all sectors should be subject to potential consideration for competitive bidding (ECJ 2005a; 2005b; European Commission 2006c). The policy conclusion from this is that, for example, all local government procurement should be subject to the consideration of interest in the context of internal markets, also below the given threshold limits and within sectors not included within the scope of the directive. This has implications to the ways in which local government funded, but contracted-out services, are procured. In Finland, Treaty of the European Union provisions were used to justify the inclusion of health services within government procurement law in Finland (see Chapter 8).

The European Union Working Time Directive has been a sticky point between the United Kingdom and the European Union, but has been raised in particular in the context of NHS and junior doctors. The directive regulates the hours of work – working time – so as to enhance occupational health and safety. This standardises the amount of working time permitted and has a particular impact on those occupations where long hours have been the norm (such as long-distance drivers and trainee doctors). While a directive requires Member States to act in order to achieve the given results they do not strictly define the means that should be used. Treaty provisions state that a directive shall be binding, as to the results to be achieved, upon each Member State to which it is addressed, but shall leave to the national authorities the choice of form and methods (Article 249 TEC or Article 288 Treaty of Lisbon 2007).

Within the UK and subject to the agreement of the individual worker an opt-out from the regulation was possible. But the threat that the European Parliament might remove this opt-out in December 2008 has reinvigorated current debate. The issue has been further problematised by a European Court of Justice case concerning on-call time, in which on two occasions the Court has held that when a doctor is obliged to be present in a hospital or health centre this counts as working time also if he/she sleeps or rests during this time (ECJ 2000; ECJ 2003) Working Time Directive has not been a big issue for the Finnish health system as the government has remained flexible in its stance on the matter and the issue was hardly mentioned as part of our interviews (Eduskunta 2008). While the Working Time Directive clearly re-inforced the message that European Union processes can affect national health systems, the impacts are also related to overall policies in relation to working time and the protection of workers.

Health systems-related measures do not only emerge within the mandate of DG Sanco. Health and social issues were initially under DG Employment, with responsibilities both for health and social policies. 'Services of general economic interest' have been a particular area of the DG Employment and this has lead to contestation between the otherwise relatively weak direc-torates in the Commission. The new contribution on services of general inter-est has also been combined with the more single market orientated citizens' agenda (European Commission 2006d; 2007b; 2007c).

In the NGO community, where a large share of nongovernmental organisa-tions in many countries are contractors and providers of services, the defin-ition of 'services of general interest' has become of broader interest, as such services are excluded from the reach of internal market rules and regulations. Considering the earlier discussed issue of services of 'general interest' as a residual category, the other aspect of this debate is that the whole European Union NGO community becomes engaged with the definition issues in respect to the 'services of general interests' with less focus on how 'services of general economic interest' are defined. The emphasis on a citizens' agenda and rights could provide a new opening in the sphere of consumer rights. However, the single market-driven emphasis becomes more problematic in relation to pharmaceuticals, where information to patients is considered part of these rights in order for patients to make the right choices (European Commission 2007c).

The role of pharmaceutical policies in the European Union is likely to increase in relevance to health systems due to two factors. First, the global corporate pressure on European Union in the context of industrial policies is significant and also reflected in European external relations and trade policies. The pharmaceutical industry has been seen, together with the biotechnology industry, as the main lobbying power within the European Union in the 1990s (Greenwood 1997). Second, the rising costs of pharmaceuticals are becoming an issue within European health systems as well as mobility of patients across countries. This is a particular issue for the new entrants to the European Union struggling with proportionally higher pharmaceutical costs. In this light the capacity of Member States to halt the rising costs of pharmaceuticals becomes vulnerable, particularly if the European Union emphasis remains strongly within industrial policies and policy priorities.

Pharmaceutical policies are dealt within the DG for Enterprise and Industry, which sets the basic framework for the area. While it was hoped that the establishment of the Pharmaceutical Forum would improve and strengthen the role of health concerns in the area, the results of this process have been limited. The pharmaceutical package was released on 10 December 2008 with the title *Safe, Innovative and Accessible Medicines: A Renewed Vision for the Pharmaceutical Sector* (European Commission 2008c). One of the crucial disagreements on the issue has been the case for 'corporate information sharing' on prescription medicines directly to patients, where traditional views have considered this as advertising and not appropriate practice within the European Union due to the conflicts of interests and experiences in the nature of information sharing in the area.

The current efforts need to be understood in relation to the promotion of direct-to-consumer-advertising of prescription drugs, which is currently prohibited within Europe. The importance in this context is that rather than contributing to neutral and more objective sources of consumer information or to measures to guide patients to the sites with reliable and impartial information on the internet, the focus has been almost solely on the rights of corporations to provide information for patients on prescription drugs. This is important for demand creation in the area especially as governments are increasingly reluctant to reimburse markedly more expensive new products without evidence of major clinical benefits in comparison to existing cheaper treatments. A recent OECD study on global pharmaceutical markets also concluded that in practice few new products offer this as most are based on incremental innovation (OECD 2008).

However, the European pharmaceutical policy agenda remains strongly shaped by industry priorities and agendas reflected in the policy documents and actions (European Commission 2008c). Central aspects of their agenda include speeding up regulatory processes to get medicines earlier into the market, emphasising counterfeiting and enforcement issues in the field. There is thus a due unease over the extent to which citizen and public interests and public health considerations have been sufficiently a part of the Commission consultation process. Web-based and public Commission consultations may have resulted in the stronger representation of industry priorities than would otherwise have been the case.

Commission proposals also cover global work and interests (European Commission 2008c), where European corporate and trade policy interests are not necessarily in line with the due rights of developing countries' governments to use the TRIPS flexibilities. Because of the difficulties encountered by developing countries in using the flexibilities allowed in the TRIPS Agreement, these were further emphasised in the WTO Ministerial Conference Doha Declaration, which states that the TRIPS Agreement does not and should not prevent Member States from taking measures to protect public health (World Trade Organisation 2001). However, in practice, when governments have taken advantage of these, European trade officials have been fast to react (Mandelson 2007).

On the other hand, it is likely that public health policies could benefit more from the sectoral inquiry of the Directorate General for Competition. The initial inquiry has brought up substantial concerns over the ways in which entry of generic medicines takes place later than could be expected. The preliminary inquiry suggests that about €3 billion could have been saved in costs of medicines, should the entry have taken place without a delay. The inquiry discusses as well the ways in which defensive patenting, litigation and other measures have been used to delay generic entry (European Commission 2008c). As the sectoral inquiry will be finally reported in spring 2009, it will be of interest where the future balance in relation to public health and health policy needs, corporate and industrial policy priorities and competition-related concerns will settle.

The European Union e-health initiatives and measures are also a double-edged sword. While understood as measures to diminish healthcare costs and enhance productivity, these are also seen as an emerging area for commercial activity. Commission communication on e-health action plan presents e-health as a future growth area with prospects of covering 1 per cent of health expenditure in 2000 to up to 5 per cent of the total EU-wide health budget in 2010 (European Commission 2004d). However, what can be considered as an interesting area for commercial growth does have implications to financing of health.

While e-health has been promoted on the basis of the potential to increase productivity, the growing costs of IT within health systems do warrant careful assessment whether the promised gains do actually realise. The European Union focus on health records and cross-border interoperability needs also to be seen as a measure for the creation of true European healthcare markets, which would allow information on patients to accompany them or be accessible for them across countries and as a result enable free mobility within the

European healthcare markets (European Commission 2008d). This is a part as well of the new proposal on patient rights in cross-border care under Article 16 titled e-health (European Commission 2008a). Considering again the magnitude of estimated – and possibly overestimated – cross-border care taking place currently, the process towards interoperability has to be driven by other needs than merely tackling cross-border care as such.

Services directive and expansion of the competence of DG Health

The extension of internal market rules to health gives two benefits for the DG Sanco in terms of, first, giving scope for articulation of stronger European Union presence on health so as not to let the European Court of Justice lead the European Union health policies and in particular health services in relation to Member States. Second, emphasising the legitimacy of internal market regulations within the European Union gives a stronger power position from which DG Sanco can argue in relation to issues towards the Member States without being challenged on the basis of competence and subsidiarity. Furthermore, in comparison to public health issues, there is substantially more money and financial interests in health services, which are relevant to position and power within the Commission. It is in this context understandable – though not preferable – that DG Sanco has taken this route in the area. On the other hand this creates a problematic combination for the Member States, which assume that strengthening health within the European Union would provide a counterforce to internal market pressures, rather than another force conveying these pressures to the Member States.

The services directive, initially launched by the DG internal market, was a political choice. It can also be argued that it was based on commercial prospects on trade in services, rather than on the rights of the individual patients which had taken their cases to the European Court of Justice. However, in the context of the European Union the emphasis on citizens' interests and rights has given this concern further clout. The arguments concerning the need to consider health within the health policy arena rather than internal markets was strongly promoted by the nongovernmental community and, as opposition to inclusion of health services was seen as an obstacle to the approval of the whole directive, it was shifted to a separate directive to be proposed by DG Sanco.

DG Sanco had been active in expanding its remit beyond public health. It almost succeeded in changing the relevant article in the context of the proposed new Constitutional Treaty, but as this failed to be ratified, DG Sanco has had to rely on more incremental steps such as a consultation on health services, emphasising mobility of patients to create a broader health strategy. This expansion has also been reflected in the title of the Commission's public health programme that has now been changed to a health programme creating more scope for measures with respect to health services. The DG Sanco managed health services directive was initially leaked broadly during autumn

2007, to the extent that according to the NGO community it might have been the most broadly leaked document in European Union history. However, it was postponed, allegedly for the purpose of not disturbing the process of approval of the revised Constitutional Treaty, which was proceeding again in spring 2008, including decisions made within the United Kingdom on the approval of the new proposed reform treaty.

The new health service directive, while emphasising patient rights in the title, is still predominantly about adjusting health systems operations to follow internal market rules. This is reflected in the fact that patient rights are not specifically addressed within the aim or scope of the proposal, which has its focus on cross-border healthcare (European Commission 2008a). This is understandable as also in the earlier versions of the directive the title was 'on safe, high-quality and efficient cross-border healthcare'. The existing cooperation in the context of social security (Regulation 1408/71) covers the cases with respect to tourists, pensioners and temporary workers abroad as well as when Member States send patients abroad, even for treatment which is not available in the current system. However, in this context the new directive focus is more on scope and possibilities of people to seek healthcare in another Member State. It is also likely that some references to services will be taken out from the actual directive as a result of negotiation with European Parliament and European Council (European Parliament 2008a). Some changes seem to have taken place also due to conflicting interests of DG Employment in the context of services of general interest. The directive is based on the free movement of patients and services, but not on free movement of health professionals.

The main concern for many Member States seems to have been related to the stipulations concerning pre-authorisation requirements and more specifically when this is to be allowed. The Commission solution has been to add a condition – a rather unclear one concerning financial sustainability – which on the basis of the impact assessment is unlikely to be ever fulfilled.

It is expected that as result of the feedback from the European Parliament and European Council the proposal will be changed if not abandoned. However, it is also likely that a slightly modified version proceeds due to the focus on the minor numbers of cross-border care assuming limited relevance for the proposal. On the other hand, it is possible that the very purpose of this proposal is to set health services in the context of internal market regulatory framework on the basis of Article 95 of the Treaty of the European Union with a focus on functioning of internal markets, which is explicit in the recital part of the directive. The implications for subsidiarity and competence in health services-related issues are therefore a more important aspect of the same discussion.

Finally, the role of the European Union in international health work is to be strengthened and has been included as part of the new health strategy and policy mandate in the new health strategy (European Commission 2007b). European Member States already coordinate a large share of their international activities; however, in the field of pharmaceutical policies and health services-related matters this is not a straightforward matter due to direct conflicts of interest (see Chapter 4).

There is a risk that the European Union policy stance on pharmaceutical policies internationally represents the interests of European industries in a way that compromises global public health or even national public health.

European Union, citizens and public involvement

The European Union's influence on citizens and public involvement takes place through different avenues. One aspect of these is that of traditional democratic accountability through Member State governments and the European Parliament, whose role is limited, but at times an essential form of influence. It is also tied to the introduction of constitutional treaties and the difficulties in their adoption, as citizens have turned these down on the basis of popular votes. This has implications to the legitimacy of the European Union as well as to the expanding set of agendas. As European Community history and background has been based on arrangements for common markets, these structures have not been and are not geared towards conveying democratic accountability and representativeness as such. It is also this context that frames the role and relevance of public involvement, citizens and participation at the European level.

The main formal route in relation to participation seemed to emerge through the consideration of governance issues as part of the White Paper on Governance (2001). This paper explicitly brought up openness, participation, accountability, effectiveness and coherence as five guiding principles for all levels of governance, including European. It is articulated that the application of these five principles reinforce those of proportionality and subsidiarity. However, critical assessments have been made in particular in relation to realities of participation and the lack of addressing the issues of legitimacy and trust as real challenges to European Union governance and democratic accountability (see Joerges *et al.* 2001).

The role of European civil society networks is conveyed through formal and informal consultation processes. The traditional route to this has been consulting and administrative practices through work in committees and formal consultations mechanisms. One aspect of this is work through consumer organisations and issues as, due to the dominance of market considerations, the voice of consumers becomes more important.

One aspect of citizen action and rights is the judicial route. The court cases on patient mobility in health within the European Court of Justice could also be seen as examples of the application of the right to and for free mobility. Further possibilities could be considered in the context of the EU Charter on Fundamental Rights.

A more recently utilised and increasing route is that of interest group lobbying and engagement with 'stakeholder community'. It is important to note that reference to stakeholder groups tends to imply interest groups in practice. These have gained ground alongside a broader emphasis on participation. Thus when there is an emphasis on inclusion of stakeholders in regulatory processes, this is an issue, which takes another meaning, in relation to regulatory measures and the scope for industry influence. One recent addition to this is the inclusion of internet consultations open to all actors, which allows as well to voice demands for particular policy options and choices. In this context it is important that the Commission tends to interpret the consultation processes and set the questions asked, which then establishes the framework in which consultation is made. The European Commission also initiated a citizenship programme in 2006 (Decision 2006), whose purpose is to encourage active European citizenship and identity.

The European Commission maintains a health forum that consists of an Open Forum and a Health Policy Forum for key umbrella organisations and networks active in the area. The Commission has also enabled the establishment of a Patient Forum with patient groups and patient organisations as central actors. The Patient Forum has been criticised over the corporate engagement and financing of its member organisations (HAI 2005). Another concern in relation to nongovernmental organisations is the way in which the Commission expects shared participation in terms of results and financing on common matters. This pressure to 'share' can extend beyond the capacities of nongovernmental organisations and lead to a bias towards wealthier and interest organisation engagement.

The right to information and access to information is centrally an issue of transparency, promoted by the European Union, but remains challenging in practice. However, in the field of health, the right of corporations to provide 'information' to patients has become a political issue at the European Union level. In this context the views of patient and consumer organisations differ while European consumer representatives recommend more information for patients, they do not see the pharmaceutical industry as an appropriate source of unbiased information for consumers (BEUC 2007).

The participatory processes within the European Union machinery also create scope and spaces for policy lobbying in the context of think tanks, policy networks, seminars and cooperative efforts with the Commission. This type of activity is of concern with respect to health systems as most health NGOs have dealt mostly with public health matters as health services have not been a European Union issue. EHMA – the European Healthcare Management Association – is one of the few organisations with focus on services and which has been active over a longer period. On the other hand local governments have long had an EU office and the NHS Confederation launched an office in Brussels in 2007. In the European Parliament it has a health and consumer intergroup, whose secretariat is maintained by two nongovernmental organisations, European Public Health Alliance (EPHA) and BEUC, the European consumers' organisation.

In the field of interest group action, for example, the Swedish think tank TIMBRO's health project has been re-established as European Consumer Powerhouse with pharmaceutical industry funding and a pro-service liberalisation position. The role of participation and engagement has a different emphasis in the light of European networks with industry financing available not only to interest networks and think tanks but also to patient organisations. This issue has been raised in the critical assessments of the role and activities of patient groups (see HAI 2005; Herxheimer 2003).

Lobbying itself is not a marginal issue in Brussels. In 2007 the citizen rights and constitutional affairs department study on lobbying revealed evidence on widespread practice (Coen 2007). On the basis of a report on the matter, the European Parliament has since made a resolution, on 8 May 2008, which proposes a framework for the activities of lobbyists (European Parliament 2008b; 2008c).

Conclusion

The European Union has become increasingly focused on the realisation of the four freedoms, which are reflected in the pressure for constitutionalisation, and the changing context and interpretation of subsidiarity. This has resulted in an increasing influence of European Union policies on national policy space in relation to how health services are regulated and governed at a national level. This creates pressures on nation states for the commercialisation of health systems as well as promoting the individualisation of financing and organisation of care in order to ensure mobility across Member States.

This expansion of European Union influence takes place in the context of a shift from public health to health strategy, but also, and perhaps more importantly, in the context of the Lisbon Strategy of promoting competitiveness and the enhancement of the four freedoms as specified in the Treaty of the European Union. While an emphasis is placed on health services and services of general interest, these seem to do little to limit the European influence on national health systems in areas where commercial opportunities could be expanded.

While the European Union is expanding its role to the field of health services, the main articulation of this issue is currently in terms of patient rights. However, substantively this seems to have less to do with patient rights and more to do with internal markets regulation. The emphasis and focus on internal market regulations and the provisions of the Treaty of the European Union as the basis for legitimacy for an expanded European Union regulatory role is important to Member States and the ways in which competence over health services is shared between Member States and the European Union.

The embracing of participation at the European level is compromised due to the major involvement of interest groups and the ways in which participation mechanisms empower strong actors. Three potential avenues for the future can be envisaged. First, in terms of citizens, healthcare and markets, there is some scope for strengthening social rights through European Union activities and processes; however, it is unclear the extent to which this is likely to take place. The second, and more likely the future, is one where the joint action of economic and legal pressures moves Member States towards more individualised and market-friendly health systems. In other words the potential for health systems to address issues such as inequality become undermined by the pressure for commercialisation. The third option is that, as European treaties are not natural laws, appropriate negotiation and measures are taken to constrain European decision making and correct the current situation. Such an approach should include the reassertion of appropriate exceptions in order to ensure that European health systems can maintain the values expressed by the European Council and that sufficient European or national health policy space and resources are secured to achieve these aims.

6 England

Choice, voice and marketisation in the NHS

Contrasting with Finland and Sweden, England has a long history of health policy explicitly framed in terms of both markets and patient and public involvement. Further, there is an extensive literature critically analysing English health policy and engaging with both these sets of issues (e.g. Coulter and Magee 2003; Harrison 2004; Pollock 2004; Hogg 2008). Therefore the structure of this chapter is different and seeks to illustrate the ways these two themes have evolved and interacted in health policy over the last 20 years. We begin with a discussion of the context and broader background for policy changes and propose three distinct waves of health reform. We discuss the politics of these measures and go on to touch on the role and relevance of the European Union and globalisation before presenting some concluding reflections.

The context and background of policy changes

The British National Health Service (NHS) was founded in 1948 to provide comprehensive, universal healthcare based on need, free at the point of delivery, regardless of ability to pay. In this sense, the NHS healthcare system was designed around risk sharing, risk pooling, and the promotion of collective values over individual choice.

The organisational structure of the current NHS comprises two distinct sections: primary and secondary care. Primary care is characterised as a front-line service, facing the public, and is generally the first point of contact for patients to access medical care. Primary Care Trusts (PCTs) have overall responsibility for primary care and have a key duty in commissioning secondary care, providing community care services. PCTs oversee General Practitioners (GPs) and NHS dentists. NHS Mental Health Services Trusts provide mental healthcare in England and are overseen by the PCTs. PCTs control 80 per cent of the NHS budget, and are responsible for ensuring healthcare service provision within their area. PCTs also work with local authorities and other agencies to provide local social care. Mental health trusts provide heath and social care services through GPs and other primary care services. Care Trusts (CT) have been tasked to work across both health and social care. Despite policy ambitions, currently their numbers are relatively few.

Secondary care, or acute healthcare, comprises both elective and emergency care. Currently, thirteen ambulance trusts cover England, which provide emergency access to acute healthcare. The NHS is also responsible for providing transport to get patients to hospital for treatment. Established in 2002, Strategic Health Authorities (SHAs) are responsible for performance managing and improving and health services in their local area. NHS hospitals are managed by acute trusts, and employ a large part of the NHS workforce. Some acute trusts are regional or national centres for more specialised care, others are attached to universities and help to train health professionals. Foundation hospitals were introduced in April 2004, and are run by local managers and staff, with input from the public. Whilst they remain within the NHS and its performance inspection system, they have been allowed greater financial and operational freedom than other NHS trusts.

Reform of NHS provision in England has been complex, involving changes in supply, demand, management and transaction. These changes interact in the context of a shifting policy arena where patient and public involvement, patient choice, commissioning, competition, marketisation, and the regulation of healthcare systems vie for relative supremacy and are framed by European and broader global pressures. Central to healthcare reforms in England over the last two decades has been the application of competition within the NHS and the development of an internal healthcare market. This has involved the separation of healthcare purchaser and provider functions, the retrenchment of state provision of dentistry, opticians, and some ancillary services, and the introduction of market forces to formerly protected NHS structures. Such an approach has reinforced long standing tensions between the overlapping domains of independent and public sectors in healthcare service provision and the place of the patient as citizen or consumer or both.

The drive for greater market-led reform of the NHS was heavily influenced by neo-liberal and New Public Management arguments, whereby enhanced healthcare commodification enthymemically resolves vices in the public domain such as fiscal inefficiency, bureaucracy, and lack of accountability, with the pre-collectivist virtues of independence, self-reliance, and privacy (Hayek 1979). Citizens and patients formally subject to the vagaries of government bureaucracy and the professional paternalism of biomedicine are transformed via the market place into active, self-realised healthcare customers. In this sense, problems of accountability and efficiency are translated and settled through the introduction of a health market.

Through the translation of patient into consumer, neo-liberal political economy emphasises exit rather than voice, and replaces political relationships with market forces (Marquand 2004). The shift from a patient-centred NHS model to a market-oriented one was achieved via a linguistic turn which transformed the patient into a consumer; the rhetoric of civil society is subsumed by one of individual choice. The evolution of patient choice via patient-focused care in the context of informed consent claimed to equalise power differentials between health experts and the community. There exists, however, a conflict between the collective value of the public or greater good and the practice of participatory engagement in healthcare provision in the limited form of individual choice concerning the location of treatment. As Callaghan and Wistow note, 'the difficulties involved in exercising rights in relation to welfare goods have long been recognised' (2006: 585).

Economic efficiency and increased productivity are central to health reform but NHS healthcare policy reform has emphasised the importance of 'rights and responsibilities'. This linkage emerged in the Conservative government's Patient's Charter (Department of Health 1991). More recently, New Labour's modernisation agenda further deployed this device to link elements of both the marketisation and involvement imperatives. In turn, this discourse broadens and emerges through the dual strands of collective engagement and competition, characterised by the continuing tension between the 'choice' and 'voice' agendas. This tension is also reflected in debates over the location of power. The trend for healthcare reform to centralise power and limit autonomy has been met by a localisation agenda that promotes responsiveness to local communities and the personalisation of care. Note, the policy shift to 'decentralisation' (see Burns *et al.* 1994), in practice, involved both the devolution of responsibility to hospital trusts and the opening up of healthcare provision to greater mixed economy of care.

Whilst the introduction of the internal market in 1991 led to a radical reformation of the relationship between the state and the National Health Service and sought to harness competition, there also has been a long-standing history of patient and public involvement (PPI) in the NHS since the early 1970s. In this context Milewa *et al.* (2002) have identified four discrete PPI periods during this timeframe:

1 Pre 1974, where community involvement in healthcare devolved to elected representation from municipal authorities and lay membership on hospital committees and boards.
2 From 1974–1990, Community Health Councils were established and developed, foregrounding elements of the involvement agenda; involvement tended to be conceptualised as consumer feedback.
3 During 1990–1997, the rhetorical attachment to patients' rights and responsibilities advanced the involvement agenda but achieved relatively modest gains in practical terms.
4 Post 1997, PPI became a central plank of both healthcare policy rhetoric and operational structures.

To which we add a fifth period:

5 Post 2003, where rhetorical policy ambitions for collaborative democracy were characterised by the attempted integration of the seemingly divergent imperatives of involvement and consumerism as dual drivers for healthcare service improvement and local responsiveness.

In this sense, in attempting to synthesise and re-integrate the potentially divergent trajectories of 'voice' and 'choice', New Labour has sought to make a case for public service improvement and the consequence of improved services as co-produced and a shared responsibility.

In terms of healthcare policy the two streams, of involvement and marketisation, have been interwoven and their trajectories intersect. We propose that this intersection could be conceptualised as three waves of reforms that have deployed both of these seemingly divergent drivers in order to improve services. Critically, whilst the deployed mechanisms have not been significantly different, they have been presented and justified in very different, often oppositional terms.

The first wave of reforms brought the introduction of the internal market, focused on mechanisms to contain healthcare costs and coincided with neo-liberal inspired reforms that swept OECD countries. The second wave can be tied to the New Labour government that came to power in 1997 and highlighted patient and public involvement as well as consumerism and competition to leverage quality improvement across the NHS. The third wave of reforms, emerging in early 2001, twinned patient and public involvement and patient choice to further a localism agenda and promote an NHS that was responsive to locally expressed needs – whether expressed through individual choice or collective voice. In the following sections we describe the rhetorical policy moves that underpin these waves of reform in order to unpack their practical implications.

The first wave: the evolution of involvement and the introduction of the internal market

Whilst improved efficiency rather than enhanced democracy may be the core driver for participation (Bang 2004), the enhancement of the role of local accountability in healthcare can be viewed as an attempt at reconciling issues-based politics with collective wellbeing. The pressure for greater patient and public involvement (PPI), or 'voice', from outside healthcare was prompted by the desire to move away from an NHS seen as a bureaucratic expert system driven by medical concerns and delivered through patterns of paternalism. PPI was seen as an opportunity to reconcile collective responsibility, ties of mutual obligation, and consensus with the imperatives of efficiency, accountability, and centralised control and create a dialogue between the situated 'lived experience' of healthcare professionals and local stakeholders. Here, the political voice of the collective (Williams 1998) would provide an antidote to corporate and clinical governance and endow it with accountability that emerged from shared community governance.

PPI in England first evolved at a local level as Patient Participation Groups were established in 1972 in Berinsfield, South Oxford. The working practices of these groups were built on trust and goodwill, based on co-production and evolving relationships. These local structures resulted in the formation of the

National Association for Patient Participation that remains the central voluntary sector organisation focused on involvement in primary care.

Community Health Councils (CHCs) were established in 1974 in order to strengthen community 'voice' within NHS structures and monitor local services as part of the NHS Reorganisation Act 1973. CHCs were a dramatic departure from previous medically dominated approaches and were initially seen as successful but weak (Klein and Lewis 1976; Hallas 1976). CHCs had relatively limited powers, operated with small budgets and had limited access to information and key meetings. The Councils were organised to be independent of Area Health Authorities but funded by District Health Authorities. From the beginning they were very varied in their impact but often found it difficult to challenge institutional decisions, and came to be perceived as having difficulties in adequately representing diverse range of local constituencies.

The relationship between this early incarnation of PPI, their national body the Association of Community Health Councils of England and Wales, and the policy-making community was characterised by a certain ambivalence; successive governments tended to distrust 'bottom-up' challenges to institutional decision-making processes. Perhaps this explains why CHCs were acknowledged to be relatively politically underpowered, with limited legal, resource, and information bases (Baggott 2004). In part this was because they were subject to different visions not only locally but at a national political level.

> The original Conservative vision was of the CHC as a local consumer group, who would make representations to health authorities on behalf of local residents about detailed aspects of the local delivery of services. They did not want CHCs to become involved in policy or be in any way political. The Labour vision was more ambitious. They wanted CHCs to strengthen democracy in the health service, and to take on professionals and help implement national policies at local level.
>
> (Hogg 2008: 30)

Thatcherite Conservative policy healthcare reforms of the 1980s and 1990s were characterised by increased moves towards enhanced private sector competition, with patients largely conceptualised as consumers (Baggott 2004). These moves were underpinned by a marketisation imperative based around the three 'e's of economy, efficiency and effectiveness, and a subsequent democratic rationalisation comprising the two 'r's of rights and responsibilities (Orme *et al.* 2001).

The rhetoric underpinning the radical reform of NHS structures under Health Ministers Waldegrave, Bottomley and Dorrell emphasised the efficient deployment of resources in order to better control public expenditure. Throughout the 1980s, the deployment of new public management theory, characterised by this rhetoric of efficiency, was operationalised via requirements to generate savings, the introduction of performance indicators, cost-effective ancillary service audits, the launch of income-generation initiatives, and Rayner scrutinies.

The seminal Griffiths Report (Griffiths 1983) marked the rise of 'new managerialism' in the NHS under the Thatcher government. Promoting a business-inspired new approach to healthcare, Sir Roy Griffiths, a managing director of the supermarket chain Sainsbury's, diagnosed institutional stagnation as a malaise located within the organisational structure of the NHS. The remedy prescribed was a dynamic drive for greater efficiency and, hence, productivity.

> Down the tatty corridors of the NHS, new and dedicated heroes would stride – the general managers. Inspired by their leadership a new sort of staff would arise. Armed with better information and new techniques from the private sector, much more closely monitored yet working as a team, they would at last take collective pride in their work – and responsibility for it.
>
> (Strong and Robinson 1990: 3)

The NHS and Community Care Act (1990) took effect in 1991 for hospital care and in 1993 for social care, with a new GP contract introduced from 1990. Harrison (2004: 33) describes the reforms as having four core elements:

1   the separation of purchasers and providers of hospital services
2   the reorganisation in to semi-autonomous organisational forms (*trusts*) of hospitals, ambulance services and community social services
3   the opportunity for GP practices to be relatively autonomous purchasers of health services for the patients as *fundholders*
4   the integration of health service sectors.

The reforms led to a system of rounds of audited performance review and evaluation based on specified sets of objectives and targets delivered by new tiers of managers. Post-Griffiths Report health policy tended to bolster managerial rather than medical power. However, Griffiths did propose the 'cogwheel' system, whereby healthcare professionals involved themselves in decision-making processes concerning priority-setting and resource use. Nevertheless, the evolution of a decision-making structure based on political and ministerial power and replacing the more consensual historic approach presaged further divisions.

Working for Patients (Department of Health 1989) was a deeply contested document, both in the political and NHS arenas, since it attempted to precipitate change from a medical to a market model, from healthcare professional and patient to service provider and consumer. Further, it began a shift in governance and accountability from a medically led system dominated by the demands and expectations of physicians premised on the hospital as the main source of healthcare, to a service driven by managers within a centralised framework of targets where the planning, prioritisation and 'purchasing' of healthcare services was separated from their provision. This 'market', however, was driven not directly by patients purchasing services with their funds but indirectly within a 'quasi-market' (Le Grand and Bartlett 1993).

> A quasi-market is like a market in the sense that there are independent providers competing for custom within it. But it differs from a normal market in at least one key way. This is that users do not come to a quasi-market with their own resources to purchase goods and services, as with a normal market. Instead the services are paid for by the state, but with money following users' choices.
>
> (Le Grand 2007: 41)

An unintended consequence of the adoption of this enhanced market-based system was the alteration of the relationship between healthcare professionals and patients. In this sense, decisions were to be driven by consumer demand, rather than provider judgement. Paradoxically, *Working for Patients* also centralised ministerial decision-making powers. Thus the new centralised objective setting and review mechanisms were in tension with the autonomy and accountability in the new trusts at the local level.

Working for Patients developed the theme of customer orientation in the context of consumer rights later rehearsed in the *Patient's Charter* (Department of Health 1991). The twinned rhetorical policy imperatives of 'choice' and 'voice' were conjoined in order to 'give patients, wherever they live in the UK, better healthcare and greater choice of the services available' (Department of Health 1989: 3). The White Paper went on to stress that it was important to 'make the Health Services more responsive to the needs of patients' via the delegation of 'as much power and responsibility as possible ... to the local level' (Department of Health 1989: 4).

On balance, the *Patient's Charter* (Department of Health 1991) clearly defined patients as consumers and effectively embedded new public management within the NHS. But the Charter also recognised contrasting imperatives. As the Director of King's Fund noted at the time,

> [T]he patient's charters recognise the importance of public services, a welcome change from the past decade. It also emphasises that the NHS belongs to the public, which has a right to know what to expect. Giving patients more power is not stated explicitly, but the charter should help to achieve this.
>
> (Stocking 1991: 1148)

Drawing on the rhetoric of patients' rights, the Charter attempted to implement *Working for Patients* by setting out certain 'rights' and standards of healthcare provision, emphasising the role of individual patient-consumer rights in the context of service provision at both national and local levels. However, since these 'rights' did not have mandatory force and thus could not be guaranteed, rather than provide enforceable rights, it raised expectations by setting out a range of aspirational standards, and only suggested means of complaint (Tritter 1994).

The Charter also gave effect to the quasi-internal, managed or 'mimic' market for NHS services based on Enthoven's efficiency and responsiveness argument (Enthoven 1985). This was a key move since the internal market acted as private sector market mechanism entry point to healthcare service provision. However, this drive for greater efficiency through the introduction of enhanced market mechanisms did not prove entirely successful. This is because, whereas formerly integrated NHS systems were dependent on risk pooling, risk sharing, cost sharing and hence low transaction costs, the quasi-market resulted in quasi-pricing allied to the increased cost of these 'negative externalities'. Also there existed political sensitivities associated with the potential end-product of intra-hospital competition – the possible failure of the least competitive organisations.

The gap in taking forward substantive patient and public involvement was finally broken with the publication of *Local Voices* (NHSME 1992). This document discussed the value of enhanced incorporation of community knowledge and views within NHS structures. Presented as a challenge to service purchasers to involve local communities in priority-setting decision-making processes, *Local Voices* also encouraged local authorities to consult their communities about the overall form of local healthcare service provision. However, Paton judged that 'the language of consumerism was used to justify an increasing stress upon market . . . *Local Voices* was more about communication of the inevitable to the public than about participatory purchasing' (2000: 13).

From the mid 1990s, successive governments began to signal a shift in policy towards a greater emphasis on enhanced patient and public involvement in healthcare. Building on previous central government policy statements (NHSME 1992; Health Committee 1995; NHSE 1995), the NHS Executive (1995) made explicit policy reference to involvement, noting that 'there should be greater voice and influence given to NHS service users and carers, the development and definition of local service standards, and NHS policy at local and national level'.

Later on, the Calman and Hine report (1995) foregrounded the need for greater meaningful involvement of users in planning cancer services (see Gott *et al.* 2002). This represented an important watershed in PPI, in so far as many subsequent policy initiatives made clear reference to the user involvement aspect of the Report.

The Conservative government continued this intermittent championing of the involvement agenda throughout the remainder of their time in power. In 1996 Stephen Dorrell presented the White Paper *Primary Care Delivering the Future* (Department of Health 1996), which included patient and carer information and involvement as an emerging element of the Conservative government healthcare agenda. This was followed by *Patient Partnership: Building a Collaborative Strategy* (Department of Health and NHS Executive 1996) and the *Priorities and Planning Guidance for the NHS* (NHS Executive 1996), which was designed to give greater voice and influence to users of NHS services and their carers, and was explicit in promoting PPI by setting a medium term priority to:

> [G]ive greater voice and influence to users of NHS services and their carers in their own care, the development and definition of standards set for NHS services locally and the development of NHS policy both locally and nationally . . . Health Authorities should have a strategic plan for, and be engaged in early systematic and continuing communication and consultation with local people, users and carers' groups, community health councils and other representatives and voluntary groups, about plans to respond to local health needs and to developing local services. They should be able to demonstrate the impact of that consultation on their own plans and how its outcome has been fed back to the local community.
>
> (NHSE Executive 1996)

The attempt to formalise PPI policy by proposing a set of key aims including the promotion of users' involvement in their own care, encouraging informed choice, making the NHS more responsive to the needs and preferences of service users, and supporting effective involvement of users was invoked by health authorities and trusts but had little impact on their operating priorities (Jordan *et al.* 1998). Instead users' views were used selectively by NHS managers to justify and legitimate their own decisions and imply a community facing health authority (Harrison and Mort 1998).

Harrison sums up the impact of the reforms suggesting that they,

> contributed to an ongoing trend toward centralization of governmental control over health system actors. NHS managers came under tighter fiscal and operational control from the DOH and the NHS executive, while managerial constraints on hospital physicians also intensified. Patient and public representatives lost direct access to NHS decision channels, but fundholding and the Patient's Charter made hospitals more sensitive to some of the patients' needs.
>
> (Harrison 2004: 73)

Whilst the government was willing to allocate greater resources to the NHS and real spending grew over the period 1989–1996 (Harrison 2004: 35), at the same time pressures emerged for greater operating efficiency savings and centralised control through the development of a target-driven system. It is also worth noting that rather than improving opportunities for patient choice the quasi-market reforms tended to effectively reduce them by, among other reasons, limiting GP referral access to specialists (Holland and Fotaki 2006).

Despite the explicit statements promoting the patient and public involvement agenda, the central driver of the first wave of reforms was the containment of healthcare costs achieved through investment in a different organisational structure and the provision of incentives to deliver services that reduced waiting lists particularly for surgery (Appleby *et al.* 2003). In these terms, choice and, hence, the right of 'exit' implied diverse service delivery provisions predicated on equal access to information. However, in terms of greater democratic accountability or improved effectiveness, not only was there no convincing evidence of increased patient and public involvement at local level there was also no convincing evidence that greater competition increased productivity by hospital trusts (Hamblin 1998).

The second wave: choice and involvement to improve quality

Early New Labour rhetoric made clear allusions to the inconsistencies inherent in neo-liberal marketisation processes, and rehearsed an ideological commitment to historic communitarian Labour values. As Tony Blair noted:

> People are not individuals in isolation from one another but members of a community and society who owe obligations to one another as much to themselves and who depend on each other, in part, at least, to succeed.
>
> (Blair 1996: 5)

This theme was taken up in the White Paper *The New NHS: Modern, Dependable* (Department of Health 1997) which made explicit reference to the involvement agenda, noting that 'the health service will measure itself against the aspirations and experiences of its users' (ibid.: 66), and identified six core principles, including the need 'to make the delivery of healthcare . . . a matter of local responsibility', in order to 'rebuild public confidence in the NHS as a public service, accountable to patients, open to the public, and shaped by their views' (ibid.: 11).

The White Paper introduced PPI in service planning and priority setting, and set out an agenda for the establishment of Primary Care Groups in England, Local Healthcare Committees in Scotland, and Local Health Groups in Wales. Each Group was to be governed by a multi-stakeholder, multi-agency Board including a 'community member'. However, further demands from the British Medical Association and the General Medical Services Committee secured a Board composition where GPs' interests were dominant. Whereas the White Paper stressed the importance of multi-stakeholder debate concerning the form and function of Primary Care Trusts, the structural power differentials between stakeholder groups resulted in an unbalanced and variable outcome: 'it quickly became clear to us that some stakeholders had more impact than others, and the health authorities varied in their willingness to facilitate real debate' (Smith and Sheaff 2000: 130). In this sense, the emergence of a relative hierarchy of influence in the healthcare decision-making process, based on a particular conceptualisation of stakeholder involvement, tended to characterise early New Labour forays into PPI healthcare policy.

The idea that the patient's voice did not sufficiently influence provision of services was rehearsed in the next White Paper *Saving Lives: Our Healthier Nation* (Department of Health 1999b), which explicitly recognised the role of local community expertise within the healthcare decision-making process, and encouraged health authorities, local communities, primary care groups and primary care trusts to make use of NGOs in delivering programmes. To this end an Advisory Forum of non-governmental Public Health Organisations was established, Health Impact Assessment was applied to policy development and implementation, and the Expert Patient Programme was founded (Department of Health 2001b). The White Paper proposed an integrated 'third way' healthcare structure at individual, community and governmental levels. As Blair suggested in the Foreword, 'Individuals taking action for themselves and their families are central to this. Communities working together can offer real help' (Department of Health 1999b: i).

Patient and Public Involvement was also seen by the government as a lever to improve services by putting people in the position of monitoring services. In part to illustrate the government's commitment to involvement, the 'biggest ever listening exercise' (see Hogg 2008) was launched in May 2000. The role of the exercise was ostensibly to inform the subsequent *NHS Plan: A Plan for Investment, a Plan for Reform*, which acknowledged the lack of patients 'voice' in healthcare structures, noting that 'too many patients feel talked at, rather than listened to. This has to change' (Department of Health 2000: 88). The White Paper expressed a significant shift in the NHS and attempted to redress the perceived lacuna in patient and public 'voice' by setting out a new relationship between government and the NHS, and between the NHS and patients by proposing fundamental reforms in order to 'bring patients and citizens into decisions at every level . . . and enhance and encourage the involvement of the citizen in redesigning the health service from the patient's point of view' (Department of Health 2000: 95).

In response, the Health and Social Care Act 2001 operationalised the policy shift highlighted in *The NHS Plan* (2000). The centrepiece of this new shift was Section 11 which placed a duty on all NHS organisations (including Strategic Health Authorities, Primary Care Trusts, and NHS Trusts) to make arrangements to involve and consult patients and the public in service planning and operation, and in the development of proposals for change. The Act extended the powers of local authority elected members to review and scrutinise local health arrangements by establishing Local Authority Health Overview and Scrutiny Committees. The core rationale for the Act was to 'ensure democratic accountability to elected community representatives so that patients and the public have a voice which will have to be listened to in the future' (Lammy 2002).

Further, the NHS Reform and Healthcare Professionals Act (2002) abolished Community Health Councils and split their roles and responsibilities between a number of new structures in order to implement PPI in the NHS. The new organisations included the Independent Complaints Advocacy Service, the Commission for Patient and Public Involvement in Health, a Patient Advice and Liaison Service (PALS) and a Patients' Forum (later renamed Patient and Public Involvement Forums) within every NHS Trust. Patient and Public Involvement Forums were intended to monitor and review services in the trust they were attached to and had the power to inspect any premises, monitor the effectiveness of the PALS and ICAS in their area and elect a non-executive director to sit on their local NHS Trust board.

The Act also established a Citizens Council to advise the National Institute for Health and Clinical Excellence (NICE), set up a 'one-stop-shop' guidance facility for patients, established local authority Overview and Scrutiny Committees, introduced an annual patient survey programme, and required NHS Trusts and PCTs to publish an annual Patient Prospectus to demonstrate the relative effectiveness of their PPI strategies.

The existing 180 Community Health Councils were replaced with 572 Patient and Public Involvement Forums each made up of 12–20 appointed local people, recruited by the Commission for Patient and Public Involvement in Health (CPPIH) set up by the NHS Reform and Healthcare Professionals Act. CPPIH performance managed the Forums but also had a broader remit to employ staff to support the forums (Forum Support Organisations) and promote PPI in the NHS. At a national level Harry Cayton was appointed in 2002 as the first National Director of Patient Experience and Public Involvement, the PPI Czar.

Despite this clear policy adherence to greater 'voice' in healthcare, Coulter and Magee (2003) argue that a shift in public expectations about healthcare occurred; patients increasingly pursued the role of consumers of healthcare services by emphasising autonomous individual 'choice'. This reflects Dahl's (1961) earlier discussion on pluralist theory, which implies diffuse dispersal of power to a range of groupings through 'choice', or expressed preference, as a true analogue for interest. As Coulter points out,

> When patients are given the opportunity to make informed choices, they usually welcome it. Unreasonable or irrational demands are not as common as many clinicians fear. Patients often prefer more conservative and cheaper treatments than their doctors are inclined to recommend. Shared decision-making could be one of the best ways to ensure more appropriate uses of healthcare resources.
>
> (Coulter 2002: 47)

Although New Labour's early policy discourse is differentiated from a new-public management ideology, some argue that the 'third way' modernising agenda seemed rather similar in practice (Stewart 2003). This is because attempts to co-opt and synthesise elements of conservative ideology potentially resulted in its further deployment (Fielding 2003). In this sense, early New Labour healthcare policy tended to co-opt the mechanisms applied by the Conservative government in attempting to drive greater economic efficiency and adopted a reforming stance in relation to 'bottom-up' involvement. As Harrison notes,

> The Blair government modified or abandoned many of the NHS' market mechanisms, including fund-holding, and favoured an ethos of cooperation instead of competition . . . Despite this move away from reliance on the market and the private sector, the Blair government retained the contracting process and private finance of hospital construction.
>
> (Harrison 2004: 83)

The justification for this process was different from the Conservatives and not framed in terms of increased efficiency or productivity but rather focused on improving the quality of healthcare.

The Kennedy Report of the Public Inquiry into Children's Heart Surgery at the Bristol Royal Infirmary (Department of Health 2001b) provided a damning, powerful analysis and critique of the organisational culture of the NHS during this period. The recommended antidote was greater patient involvement, openness and transparency concerning clinical performance. Kennedy's approach advocated a shift in emphasis from clinical to managerial power, questioned the culture of clinical freedom in context of resource constraints, but left open how best to implement this shift in the decision-making processes.

This agenda supported increased managerialism to improve the quality of healthcare and responded to systemic patient safety issues allied to greater surveillance framed in terms of clinical governance, which was centrally driven, and often coerced or at least incentivised. The implementation of the Quality Outcomes Framework for GPs is an excellent example of this process and was introduced as part of the General Medical Services Contract in 2004. As the NHS Confederation and NatPaCT (2003: 4) noted at the time, 'the Quality and Outcomes Framework aims to implement current clinically-proven interventions, which should be applied across the health service to make it patient-centred and efficient'. The intention was to provide an incentive for GPs to adopt best practice by awarding points across four domains: clinical, organisational standards, patient experience and additional services.

Drawing on the Wanless Report, the strategy paper *Building on the Best: Choice, Responsiveness and Equity in the NHS* (Department of Health 2003a) attempted to consider the main themes that emerged from the *Choice, Responsiveness and Equity* consultation (Department of Health 2003c). The strategy paper functionally expanded the reach of 'choice' to encompass healthcare service provision for emergency care, children's services, mental health, maternity services, primary care, and care for the aged. In the Foreword, John Reid attempted to resolve problems associated with resource allocation and efficiency through the mechanism of enhanced choice, noting that: 'The question of resources and capacity is inextricably linked to the question of choice' (Department of Health 2003a: 4).

This imperative was rehearsed in Milburn's *Choices for All* speech to NHS Chief Executives, which discussed 'choice' as a core tenet of the government's approach to healthcare. Milburn set out, in some detail, New Labour's belief in the role that enhanced choice could make to underpinning drives for 'devolution', 'democratisation', and 'diversity', concluding that:

> I believe we can open up more choices to NHS patients. The issue is firstly, whether we should and secondly, how we could. It is often argued that capacity constraints mean that choice on the NHS is not possible .... It is certainly true that choice can only grow as capacity grows. What is not true is that some capacity is not already available or that more cannot be grown ... The main argument against more choice has been that it will bring less equity. I want to argue the reverse: that greater choice can mean greater equity ... by making choice more widely available on the NHS ... it is extended to the many not just the few. Some say poorer people do not want to exercise choice or are not able to do so. I disagree profoundly. That is patronising nonsense ... by linking the choices patients make to the resources hospitals receive ... we can provide real incentives to address under-performance in local NHS services. As we know poorer performance is often concentrated in poorer areas. Giving people the power to choose between services will drive standards up. In this way, greater choice can enhance equity, not diminish it.
>
> (Milburn 2003)

Although primarily concerned with education matters, David Miliband's 'choice and voice in personalised learning' speech to the OECD Conference on the Future of Public Sector Reform can be read as a more generalised discourse on the nature of New Labour's rhetorical stance on 'choice' and 'voice' in the context of public sector governance. Here, Miliband refers to Piore and Sabel (1986) and argues that,

> Until recently, the debate in the UK has been polarised into an argument between advocates of market solutions and those who favoured a planned approach. Our purpose in Government is to provide a new choice for those who are not satisfied to rely solely on the state or the market.
>
> (Miliband 2006: 23)

Critical commentary on the relative success of these policy interventions have been mixed: although Goes (2004) suggests that New Labour first emphasised more traditional 'communitarian' roots, and Coote notes that stakeholder engagement and empowerment were 'a crucial dimension of New Labour's efforts to forge a fresh approach to social policy that differs from the old "statist" model of the post war era and the market model of the Thatcher and Major years' (2006: 55); Baggott argues that dissatisfaction with healthcare service provision was conceptualised by the government as a rationale for embracing and extending the 'consumerist' model via greater responsiveness to patient needs and preferences (Baggott 2004).

Prior to 2004 the Labour government had increased investment but tied funding to further centralisation of power and surveillance to promote quality. In part this was a response to a series of high-profile failures in patient safety. The same mechanisms of competition, growing individual choice and patient and public involvement were used to increase transparency and promote change. The radical change in patient and public involvement establishing PPI Forums and dismantling the Community Health Councils after a track record of almost thirty years was an experiment that never had time to reach fruition. The Government actively sought to dissolve CPPIH announcing its abolition in July 2004 as part of the review of arms length bodies; PPI Forums were deemed to have never fulfilled their promise and CPPIH generated few supporters (Lewis 2005a).

The drive for greater 'voice' foreshadowed pressure for enhanced 'choice' in the context of 'local responsiveness' that would emerge in the third wave of healthcare reforms. An antecedent of this hybrid phenomenon can be found in a statement delivered by Alan Milburn to the House of Commons (18 April 2002), which conflated drivers for local accountability and greater choice. First, by noting that,

> the health service should not and cannot be run from Whitehall . . . The relationships are between the local patient and the local doctor; the local community and the local hospital. However, those relationships will not work properly until central control is replaced by local accountability.
>
> (Milburn 2002)

Milburn then goes on to conclude that 'patient choice will drive the system'. These commitments were mirrored in the then Prime Minister Tony Blair's pamphlet *The Courage of our Convictions: Why Reform of the Public Services is the Route to Social Justice* (2002) in which he conflated devolution and choice as two drivers for improvement by recommending greater choice between service providers, and increased devolved power to the front end of service delivery in order to facilitate greater local diversity and more effective consumer pressure.

The third wave: choice and involvement for local responsiveness

In the run up to the general election in 2005 the Labour Party continued to promote choice and involvement in the NHS, but the period is also characterised by a subtle shift away from quality improvement and the re-emergence of the localisation agenda, as evidenced by the *NHS Improvement Plan* (Department of Health 2004a) which set out the priorities for healthcare reform in the NHS:

> Local communities will take greater control over budgets and services ... patients and public will be given more voice in how services are planned and provided . . . In the future there will be an increasing emphasis on devolving decision-making to as near the point of delivery as possible in a partnership between commissioners, service providers and patients.
>
> (Department of Health 2004a: 73–74)

In an attempt to reinforce and reconcile 'voice' and 'choice', the public health White Paper *Choosing Health: Making Healthier Choices Easier* (Department of Health 2004b) presented involvement and consumer rights as co-produced imperatives of NHS reform, stating that whilst 'patient choice will be a key driver of the system' (Department of Health 2004b: 12), greater 'joined-up' work with a broad range of stakeholders including local communities, business and voluntary groups were necessary in order to tackle local health issues.

Drawing on the *NHS Improvement Plan* (Department of Health 2004a) the *National Standards, Local Action* planning framework (Department of Health 2004c) set out a standard-based planning framework for health and social care to be used in planning, commissioning and delivering services. The framework emphasised further devolution of decision making to local organisations, implying greater joint working and partnership between PCTs, local authorities, NHS Foundation Trusts, NHS Trusts, the independent sector and voluntary organisations. This was to be achieved, according to Sir Nigel Crisp, Chief Executive of the Department of Health and the NHS, in order to 'give the individual – the patient, service user or client – more power to improve their care and drive the whole system' (ibid.: 5).

The framework recognised the inter-dependant nature of healthcare provision, which was to be

> provided in partnership with patients, their carers and relatives, respecting their diverse needs, preferences and choices, and in partnership with other organisations (especially social care organisations) whose services impact on patient well-being.
>
> (Department of Health 2004c: 31)

The rhetorical ambition of *Creating a Patient-Led NHS: Delivering the NHS Improvement Plan* (Department of Health 2005a) was to deliver profound whole system change, emphasising both choice and involvement in order to produce a cultural change in the relationship between the NHS and both patients and the public. The Plan suggested that this cultural shift would alter the NHS from a service that 'does things to and for its patients' to one which is 'patient-led'.

In order for patient choice to influence provision, mechanisms that encouraged NHS organisations to be responsive needed to be put in place. Two policies were introduced that further elaborated the internal market: Payment by Results and Foundation Trusts.

Announced initially in 2002 (Department of Health 2002) a new system for funding was introduced from 2005. Known as Payment by Results (PbR), it comprised a prospective tariff system of payment to providers using pre-set, non-negotiable and fixed fees based on the type and number of patients treated. The price (tariff), set by the Department of Health, is the same for every provider in the country – although there is a weighting factor, the Market Forces Factor, to take account of wage differentials linked to regions (Dredge and Capaldi 2005). This mechanism created the basis for NHS Trusts to compete not only on volume but also on price and has been promoted as a mechanism to 'underpin choice' (Department of Health 2003a: 18).

The intra-trust competition resulting from this process was reinforced by the emergence of a new category of NHS organisations, Foundation Trusts (FTs). Enacted by the Health and Social Care (Community Health and Standards) Act 2003, NHS Trusts can apply to 'opt out' of central government control with greater delegation of financial powers. Foundation Trusts are presented as being more firmly tied to the local agenda as set by Members of the Foundation which are drawn from local community residents, patients and carers and trust employees (Lewis 2005b). Each Foundation Trust is answerable to a Board of Governors more than half of whom must be elected by the Members of the Foundation. Presented as a means to reinforce local responsiveness, the underpinning policy rationale for FTs concerns 'empowering patients collectively by increasing the accountability of local health services to local communities. That lies at the heart of the proposals for elected boards of NHS Foundation Trusts' (Department of Health 2003a: 13).

The idea that healthcare improvement could be co-produced via the enactment of both choice and voice set in the context of greater localisation was rehearsed in *Health Reform in England: Update and Commissioning Framework* (Department of Health 2006d), which attempted to expand the role of user involvement in healthcare provision by extending the remit of GPs, enhancing the role of patient choice in the selection of treatment site, and reforming service commissioning practices. In greater detail, the Framework aimed to allow for increased patient power and 'say' over the organisation and operation of local health services, addressed issues associated with operationalising involvement for local people through a PCT Prospectus shaped by their views, announced a means by which local communities could trigger a review of services, and attempted to facilitate greater clinician involvement through practice-based commissioning.

As if to balance any overemphasis on 'voice', *Choice Matters* (Department of Health 2006c), an update on the development of patient choice in the

NHS, focused on the experiences of patients and NHS staff, and concluded that the twin mechanisms of increased 'choice', and 'payment by results', would inexorably lead to improved service provision. Also, drawing on the *NHS Improvement Plan* (Department of Health 2004a), *Commissioning a Patient-Led NHS* (Department of Health 2005b) focused on step-changes in NHS practice-based commissioning, including functional changes in Primary Care Trusts and Strategic Health Authorities, to better reflect patient choice. This required a shift in the existing involvement structures and was one of the harbingers of the demise of PPI Forums and CPPIH.

Drawing on a wider governmental commitment to community involvement centred around the 'Together We Can' Action Plan, the *Review of Patient and Public Involvement Recommendations to Ministers from Expert Panel* sought to 'empower citizens to have more confidence and opportunities to influence public services' (Department of Health 2006a: 2). Noting that whilst some argue that an emphasis on 'choice' tends to make 'voice' redundant, the Review concluded that:

> We believe the introduction of choice makes the public voice more, not less, important . . . choice needs to be reinforced by voice particularly for the vulnerable and for those who experience health inequalities. Voice can also shape and extend the choices on offer . . . particularly for community care, and for people with disabilities and chronic illnesses. Voice is also important in its own right as it allows citizens to air their views as taxpayers.
>
> (Department of Health 2006a: 2)

An example of this stronger local voice was apparent in North East Derbyshire when a parish councillor, Pam Smith, applied for a judicial review of the way that North Eastern Derbyshire PCT awarded a general medical services contract to United Health Care without formal consultation. The judge considered that the PCT should have consulted the public under Section 11 of the Health and Social Care Act. However, he held the tendering process had been fair and that Pam Smith had not raised the matter with her local PPI forum. This was overturned on appeal where it was ruled:

> In his Lordship's view the trust was under a statutory duty to consult. It did not perform it. Mobilising the patients' forum after the decision had been taken was no remedy. It was not sufficient that if proper consultation had taken place the decision would probably have been the same.
>
> (*Smith* v. *North East Derbyshire Primary Care Trust* 2006)

This discontinuity in applying due process was compounded by one other example where a trust closed two inpatient wards at Altrincham General Hospital in March 2006 on the grounds that they were no longer safe, but did not consult on this decision. The judgement found that:

The section 11 duty to consult is of high importance. The public expect to be involved in decisions by healthcare bodies, particularly when the issues involved are contentious as they clearly were with AGH. I do not accept that the need to close the wards at Altrincham General Hospital was so urgent that it was right that no public consultation should take place. There ought to have been consultation under section 11 about the closure of the wards in so important a local provision as Altrincham General Hospital. In those circumstances I regard the decision to close the wards as unlawful and will quash.

(Trafford Healthcare NHS Trust 2006: 34)

Both of these cases illustrate ways in which individuals managed to force responses from local healthcare providers by using the legislation. In neither case, however, was the action facilitated through existing PPI mechanisms. In neither case could patient choice have been a vehicle for generating the responsiveness. The potential of further judicial recourse was increased with the passage of Section 242 (1G) of the NHS Act 2006 which strengthened the duty to consult.

In this sense, it could be argued that patient choice, while promoted by the Labour government as a mechanism for generating greater responsiveness to local needs, may not be the most effective mechanism in delivering effective service improvement. This view is supported by the Policy Commission on Public Services, *Making Public Services Personal: A New Compact for Public Services* (National Consumer Council 2004) which concluded consumers were relatively ambivalent about choice of healthcare and that patients value choice only if current healthcare providers do not meet acceptable standards.

Similarly, the National Survey of Adult In-Patients, the third in a series carried out by the Picker Institute on behalf of the Department of Health, asked almost 82,000 patients from 169 acute and specialist NHS Trusts across England about their experiences of care as inpatients. Findings suggested that 'choice' was not a priority with patients, finishing at the tail end of a list of 82 priorities. The Picker Institute noted that in comparison with other aspects of care, choice (of hospital, admission date and information pertaining to these decisions) is an issue rated low in importance by all ethnic groups.

Underpinned by the results of an Expert Panel established in 2006 the idea of a new set of structures to create and promote PPI evolved (Department of Health 2006a). The work of the Panel was foreshadowed by the Department of Health in a consultation document, *A Stronger Local Voice in the Development of Health and Social Care Services* (Department of Health 2006b), which set out the government's plans for the future of patient and public involvement in health and social care, including the establishment of Local Involvement Networks (LINks). The proposals were to encourage user and public involvement at all levels of the health and social care system by reinforcing the contextual nature of people's experience.

Established through the Local Government and Public Involvement in Health Act 2007, local authorities with social care responsibilities (County Councils and Unitary Councils) received funding (circa total £84m per year for 3 years) from the Department of Health to procure and monitor arms length 'host' organisations that help establish and support local involvement networks (LINks).

LINks are a large-scale nationally mandated, locally implemented partici- patory involvement exercise on local health and social care undertaken by the local communities, local authorities, and local PCTs (all of whom com- prise a LINk). LINks are networks of people, groups and organisations with powers relating to healthcare and social care, and are supported by a 'host' organisation to monitor and review the commissioning of local health and social care services, enter and inspect health and social care facilities, and make specific recommendations to commissioners and overview and scrutiny. The idea is to be locally flexible, to reach out and involve a broader cross section of the community, including 'seldom heard' groups. LINks are intended to impact on collective commissioning decisions, and in this sense are framed as a collective rather than an individual endeavour (representative of diversity as distinct from an aggregation of individual views).

Although LINKs have limited power to require the provision of informa- tion from local providers and commissioners, more importantly, the revised guidance on Section 242 of the NHS Act 2006 (Department of Health 2008d) stresses the significance of their involvement in commissioning services.

> Commissioners are expected to create a range of opportunities to involve users throughout the commissioning cycle. Working with the LINk is one way of obtaining their views but should not be seen as the only way to involve users.
>
> (Department of Health 2008d: 36)

This is a new departure in health policy terms as it requires NHS organisa- tions to engage with local people prospectively in the planning, prioritising and contracting of healthcare services.

LINks are an example of structures that span health and social care – the NHS and Local Government services – that have historically been separately funded and administered in England. Service improvement, community lead- ership, community empowerment, cohesion and locality working have become clear policy goals. The move towards stronger partnerships between communities, local government and the NHS is reinforced by the introduc- tion of the duty of Joint Strategic Needs Assessment. As of April 2008, pri- mary care trusts and local authorities are under a duty to work together to understand the needs of the communities they serve, informing priorities in order to 'make a real difference to health and well-being outcomes' (Department of Communities and Local Government 2007).

The government suggests that Joint Assessment provides a framework for health and local government to work in partnership with their communities to deliver choice, personalisation and empowerment to reduce inequalities, and argue that Joint Assessment will be a major tool for determining local health and wellbeing priorities. In the context of Joint Strategic Needs Assessment, Local Strategic Plans, and Local Area Agreements, it is clear that 'integrated working' practices will be important to the success of LINks and to the tranche of the New Labour modernisation agenda that conjoins choice, voice and responsiveness to local needs.

Conclusion

Two policy agendas – competition and patient and public involvement – have both been adopted to reform the organisation, governance and delivery of healthcare services in England. Over the course of the last two decades governments of different political persuasion and inclination have all found themselves relying on competition to drive change and collective involvement to legitimate significant changes in how, where and by whom healthcare services are planned purchased and provided.

The different aims apparent in the three waves of health reform we have outlined – efficiency gain, quality improvement and local responsiveness – have all been pursued using similar mechanisms – the promotion of market forces to generate competition and growing requirements to plan and justify provision to those who use the services. In some ways, patient choice serves as a point of overlap between these two very different and often competing agendas but it is far closer allied, in the guise of the individual consumer, to market mechanisms than it is to the model of responsiveness to the collective will of the people.

As Peter Beresford in the *Society Guardian* suggests:

> The choice agenda has been a failure, but empowerment will be too if it is approached in the same sloganising and superficial way. This time the government must listen to service users and their movements. They have advanced the idea of empowerment because it brings together the personal and the political. Such empowerment focuses on building people's capacity to change their lives, while helping them to work together for better public services.
>
> (Beresford 2007)

Whilst the emergence of the 'teleological discourse' of New Labour (Allen 2003) is characterised by a drive for sustained and, hence, inevitable improvement (Morrell 2006), it could be argued that a gap exists between that policy rhetoric, and the knowledge-base necessary to bring those reforms into being. The emerging discourse has emphasised a raft of concepts based around collaborative governance including involvement, participation, and capacity-building, to ensure responsiveness, and to provide policy legitimisation. However a core paradox implicit in this discourse results from the simultaneous attempt at the introduction of the conflicting imperatives of horizontal locally joined-up governance, and centralised government control – the former characterised by the emergence of drives for greater participation and localisation, the latter by the introduction of rounds of performance audits, aspirational targets, and further centralisation of power. Ham (1999) argues that this dual emphasis may be associated with the political costs of taking responsibility for difficult decisions at a central governmental level, and the diffusion of blame to the local level.

We are reminded that consumerism by itself is

> unlikely to bring about the significant improvements in the quality of care that might be achieved if the service was made directly accountable to users through community participation in decision-making, in line with local health needs. But this would involve a different view of the citizen as a member of a community, with rights and duties balanced by mutuality and control.
>
> (Calnan and Gabe 2001: 124)

This argument brings us back to the difficulty of defining and implementing policy that enables choice and voice particularly when the choice of exit is limited. The NHS, despite the continuous process of change, continues to generate overwhelming support from the public. This loyalty may hold the antidote to the potential for increased inequality linked to consumerism and greater marketisation as well as the apathy associated with involvement mechanisms that have yet to make an apparent difference, and a localism agenda that suggests little responsiveness.

Hirschman reminds us of

> The importance of loyalty . . . is that it can neutralize within certain limits the tendency of the most quality-conscious customers or member to be the first to exit . . . . As a result of loyalty, these potentially most influential customers and members will stay on longer than they would ordinarily, in the hope or, rather, reasoned expectation that improvement or reform can be achieved 'from within'.
>
> (Hirschman 1970: 79)

The fundamental issue that confronted the nascent New Labour was little different from that which confronted the Conservatives, and concerned the relative balancing of policy imperatives such as responsiveness, equity, access and efficiency (Florin and Dixon 2004). New Labour's modernising response to this challenge emerged through a series of counter-veiling moves in which 'voice' was counter-poised with 'choice' and decentralisation with greater centralisation of power and increased surveillance. A further paradox obtains: since equality of access is diminished through the erosion of comprehensiveness, and the market model implicit in 'choice' results in abandoning the historic standardised approach – the issue of how best to operationalise both 'choice', local democratic control, and community responsiveness is still evolving.

7   Sweden
A market orientation to the welfare state

In Sweden the focus and emphasis on participation and choice have been long-standing aspects of the health system. However, health policies have been shaped by other pressures and developments, and reflect the shifting priorities of the different governments. In this case study we begin with a discussion of the context and broader background for policy changes, actors and agencies involved in policy making and then go through health reform policies. We focus on citizen and patient rights and move on to discuss the politics of these measures as well as the role and relevance of the European Union and globalisation.

The context and background for policy changes

Sweden has a decentralised health system, where basic responsibilities for the provision and financing of health services are set at county councils at regional level. Medical doctors have traditionally been salaried professionals. However, different forms of reimbursement to medical doctors, such as capitation or fee-for-service, have been introduced as part of recent reforms. The financing of the health system is tax-based levied by county councils and municipalities (72 per cent in 2003) complemented by central government grants (18 per cent in 2003), user charges (3 per cent in 2003) and other sources (7 per cent in 2003). For a more comprehensive description of the Swedish health system see Glenngård et al. (2005).

In Sweden, policy changes within the health system should be seen in the context of broader governance shifts and the implementation of public sector reforms. Local government has a major role in Swedish politics and policy which has been a constituent feature of the Swedish system, and is central to the change and reform of the national healthcare system. A particular contextual issue in Sweden is the role of the 21 county councils in services provision. County councils, which were initially established as local employer organisations, by the 1960s became the legitimate mouthpiece for healthcare providers and by the 1980s had a prominent position in the Swedish health policy arena (Garpenby 1992). This shift in political power served various political interests and was in line with the broader emphasis on decentralisation and democratisation in the 1980s set within the context of public sector reforms in Sweden (Premfors 1998).

The importance of decentralisation for further reform processes is apparent in relation to deregulation. The implementation of further deregulation at a local level spurred by the free community experiments was integrated into local government legislation opening up greater scope for municipalities to organise services. The initial experiment was coordinated by the Department of Home Affairs, and led initially to conflicts between sectoral and general central government departments. During the 1980s a significant conflict emerged between the Department of Finance and the Department of Social Welfare concerning the role of private actors in delivering social welfare services (Pierre 1993).

Public attitudes towards the public sector hardened in the 1980s with an increasing percentage of the population wanting to reduce the size of the public sector (Pierre 1993). According to Saltman (1994), in the 1980s the Swedish healthcare system faced broad-based criticism emphasising a lack of focus on the needs of citizens and patients from both the political right and left. Sweden has also had a small number of medical doctors working in private practice with reimbursement from the social insurance institution. The growth of private practice in healthcare during the 1980s should be understood in the context of declining public spending on healthcare, more doctors looking for private part-time practice, increased interest in freedom of choice and willingness to pay for private care by patients as well as rising criticism of the public services (Rosenthal 1986).

In 1982 the National Health Care Act gave users the right to choose public service providers within their county council area. These rights were later expanded through an agreement between county councils and the government to include choice of primary care and secondary care specialists across both the public and private sectors nationwide (Fredriksson and Winblad 2008). However, in spite of formal 'rights to choose' there is limited understanding of the implications of choice and knowledge of its operation among health professionals (Winblad-Spångberg 2003).

The role of clients and users was also important in the context of the Swedish legislative changes within the public administration. According to Pierre (1993) the revised Public Administration Act in 1985 deviated from its predecessor mainly with respect to the rights of the client vis-à-vis the bureaucracy and gave a stronger position to clients. While decentralisation helped to ameliorate financial issues, most reforms implemented in the mid 1980s attempted to bridge the gap between the citizens and bureaucracy (Pierre 1993). Premfors (1998) has emphasised key terms during this first period of comprehensive reform defining them as 'a new public service culture', 'user influence' or 'user democracy'.

The cost of care also became an issue in the late 1980s and early 1990s with Swedish central and county governments containing health expenditures by focusing on improving costs and productivity (Twaddle 1999). This can be seen in the way the Swedish public sector reform process became dominated by these priorities leading up to the early 1990s. According to Premfors (1998) public sector reform from 1988 was run in the spirit of the Ministry of Financial Affairs and after the change of government in 1991 from a special unit within the Ministry of Financial Affairs. While public sector reform was initiated by the social democratic government, the conservative-led government elected in 1991 launched a public sector reform programme described as 'reform talk which could have been borrowed from New Zealand and the United Kingdom – and it largely was' (Premfors 1998: 151). However, its impact was not considered crucial as 'while the reform talk has certainly contained ideas of "marketisation" and "privatisation", the impact has been small, passing or almost negligible' (Premfors 1998: 158).

The emphasis on economic productivity and economic issues was further influenced by the Swedish economic crisis in the early 1990s that gave economic and financial arguments more weight. The depth of this economic crisis is apparent in that the direct costs to the taxpayer of supporting the banks through this period, by itself accounted for 2 per cent of GDP (Englund 1999). While the role of domestic and international influences, such as deregulatory measures and management in the financial sector that led to the crisis can be debated, it is clear that, while the crisis had little to do with the public sector and public services in Sweden, it dramatically changed the context and basis for managing the public sector. It is also in this context that the voice of the Ministry of Finance attained primacy. This was further strengthened as the Swedish Employers Federation and Economic Committee raised concerns over the growth of the welfare state (Ekonomikomission 1993; Twaddle 1999). This pressure was also reflected in the context of the emphasis by the Ministry of Health and Social Affairs on prioritisation and resource use (SOU 1995; 1996).

In terms of health policy making, the Swedish context in the 1980s shifted towards increasing the power of county councils and a decreasing role for central government and the national board. This suggests that in terms of policy making there was greater scope for local and regional policies within counties. In the light of the key role of county councils it is not surprising that implementation of competitive reforms in the Swedish health system began incrementally as county-level initiatives and pilot projects with substantial diversity between counties in the implementation of national programmes (Harrison and Calltorp 2000).

Since the 1980s, however, a series of medical care reforms have been implemented. While the Health and Sickness Care Law in 1982 decentralised responsibility for the medical care system to the counties and three municipalities, the 1984 Dagmar reform capped the expansion of private practice and provided greater control over state medical care expenditures through block grant funding (Twaddle 1999: 6). The multiple channels of financing in healthcare through municipal taxes, national social insurance and government subsidies were integrated and provided as a block grant based on population size. These changes were intended to manage county council expenditure; the government was now able to limit funding to county councils for healthcare, while ensuring they still retained the obligations related to service provision.

In the context of decentralisation policies, the Ädelreform in 1992 shifted care of the elderly from the responsibility of counties to local governments. The Care Guarantee (Vårdgaranti) reform in 1992 first introduced the care guarantee in Sweden; however, the introduction of care guarantee was done through negotiations between national government and county councils. The primary healthcare reform was implemented in the early 1990s. Proposals for the development of family doctors (husläkar) had been a central mission of the Liberal Party, but gained little support from the Social Democratic Party in the 1980s (Twaddle 1999). This changed when the Liberal Party came into power in 1991 and a new proposal for family doctors was presented. The legislation provided for 'free establishment' of private physicians as family physicians and provided the opportunity for citizens to change family physicians with compensation through capitation allowances supplemented by consultation and patient fees (Socialstyrelsen 1992). However, this reform was only short lived as it was repealed a year later when the Social Democrats returned to power in 1994.

In the 1990s a set of health reform initiatives was developed by the Committee on the Organisation and Financing of Medical Care, which explored different options and models, including a county model, family physician model and a model based on a national health insurance scheme (SOU 1993). The work was informed by models in other countries (SOU 1994) including interest in the NHS internal market model and more market-oriented health reforms (Whitehead *et al.* 1997). However, substantially more activity took place at the county level, where, in particular, the Dalarna and Stockholm county models have become key examples of market-model county systems incorporating purchaser–provider split. In the 1990s the government role was also reflected in work exploring the nature of cooperation with the private sector in health services provision and the promotion of plurality in service provision (SOU 1999a; 1999b; 2002).

The different responsibilities at central and local levels have become a broader concern. This was also the focus of the 'responsibility committee' – Ansvarskomitten – which emphasised regionalisation in its final report submitted in 2007. This has also been reflected in the context of hospital mergers typically prompted by potential efficiency gains (Harrison 2006). However, it is unclear to what extent these results will apply to policies under the Alliance for Sweden (a coalition of four centre-right parties), which came to power in September 2006 after 12 years of social democratic government. The current emphasis seems to be more in achieving reforms in the context of choice with legislative proposals on choice in primary healthcare and municipal services (Regeringens Proposition 2008a; 2008b).

The actors and institutional context of Swedish national health policies

In the Swedish context the role of county councils is of crucial importance for the development and implementation of Swedish healthcare policies. This is due to the strong history of local autonomy, but also the result of the developments in the 1980s as county councils strengthened their role in shaping national policies.

The role of the Swedish medical association has been important and is considered 'the only nongovernmental organisation with a seemingly major role in politically defining the problem of medical care' (Twaddle 1999: 97). However, the physicians' influence on political and policy decisions has declined since the Second World War. Medical doctors in general consider patient choice important, however, they have not been keen in promoting choice (Winblad-Spånberg 2003). In addition to the medical association representing the medical doctors, the role of nurses has been of importance. The Swedish Association for Health Professionals is the main professional and trade union organisation for nurses and midwives. From 1992 to 1993 the Association organised a critical campaign towards the health reforms and the ways in which it changed nursing practices (Blomgren 2003).

The role and relevance of other Government Ministries is reflected in the form of influence through public management reforms and emphasis on financial constraints by the Ministry of Finance. This became an issue in particular during the decentralisation process, with the Ministry of Health having difficulties adjusting to the new situation where they had less power and steering capacity at municipal and county level.

Sweden has a substantial pharmaceutical and healthcare industry that takes an active role and interest in national policies and in public contracts both within Sweden and in Europe. One example of Swedish healthcare providers is Capio, which was established in 1994, going public in 2000 and in 2008 was active in eight European countries (Capio 2008). Praktikertjänst is run in the form of a producer cooperative combining small-scale local practices within a large company providing external conditions for commercial enterprise (Praktikertjänst 2008). Third sector service providers also have their own interest organisation, Famna, which draws attention to particular aspects of health reforms relating, for instance, to the role and situation of not-for profit organisations as contractors and service providers (Famna 2008).

Swedish industry and employer associations have been active in presenting their views and have influenced healthcare reforms. The Confederation of Swedish Enterprise represents the employer associations, but services industries are also represented by Almega. Swedish industry-funded think tank TIMBRO has had a special health unit, which has since become the Consumer Powerhouse Corporation and is active at both Swedish and European levels. TIMBRO was keenly promoting, for example, the Stockholm model in the early 1990s. Government Institutes, such as NUTEK

(Swedish Business Development Agency and since 2009 the Swedish Agency for Economic and Regional Growth) as well as other research and corporate organisations are also of relevance in terms of raising issues of relevance to health policy making. NUTEK became in 2008 the basis for government measures in enhancing entrepreneurship in healthcare with an earlier programme mapping the field. The engagement of corporate sector actors and authorities has been present as well in the process of new legislative changes enabling more choice for users of health services and promoting the plurality service providers.

In health policy the role of nongovernmental organisations seems to have been divided between provider interests and presence in terms of contributing to service provision and policy-oriented lobbying efforts. The role of health or patient organisations seems to be more limited in relation to influence and decision making on broader policy aspects of service provision and reorganisation.

Healthcare reforms in the 1990s

The Swedish healthcare reforms can be seen as part of the broader context of public sector reforms and change as well as a project on their own emphasising particular changes to the health system. Blomqvist (2002) has stressed the role of ideas in national politics and of actors in taking these up. She suggests that health economists, drawing attention and introducing a 'social democrat compatible' form of healthcare reforms, and more market-oriented economists and actors, pursuing a more traditional emphasis on right-wing political parties, shaped the reform process. In the case of the former, the articulation for more market-based reforms was based on the idea of 'public competition' with 'selected market oriented mechanisms infused into the existing publicly operated delivery system' (Saltman and Otter 1987; 1992). The initial articulation also reflected the developments in the debates, discourse and politics of enhancing democracy through mechanisms of direct democracy, participation and community involvement that emphasised that public sector choice could be a mechanism to encourage civil democracy (Saltman and Otter 1989). This articulation of public competition and choice can be considered the 'soft end' of Swedish healthcare reform policy aims.

The case for reform by the more market-oriented economists was made on the basis of analysis of the costs and productivity of the health sector in the 1980s and early 1990s (Lindgren and Roos 1985; Ekonomikomission 1993; see also Bergkmark 2008; Blomqvist 2002). However, since the 1980s proportion of Swedish GDP spent on health has declined (Andersen *et al.* 2001). This decline has been to a large extent a result of economic imperatives to limit government spending, and budget controls exercised by elected county councils (Vågerö 1994). However, the high cost of care in the early 1980s and the prospects of using markets to improve this situation was clearly a contributory factor to the spread of reforms; they were seen as 'a solution' to the problem of increasing healthcare costs. The success of market-oriented reforms and patient choice in this particular aspect was problematic as costs and administrative requirements increased. In many cases the increase in costs led to abandoning the policy reforms rather than rising inequalities (see Harrison 2006).

The implementation of more market-oriented approaches was pursued by counties and applied to the new broader service provision context providing more freedom to experiment and try new provider models. Particular attention has been drawn to the Dalarna and the Stockholm models. In practice both the Dalarna and Stockholm models utilised provider–purchaser split as well as experimenting with the use of diagnostic related groups (DRGs) in hospital reimbursement (Harrison and Calltorp 2000; Garpenby 1992). The Dalarna model was initially based on a management consultancy draft with further changes made by political decision makers with the result that hospitals were defined as 'profit centres' having to attract money through contracts negotiated with the political boards responsible for the primary healthcare districts (Garpenby 1992). The Stockholm model was based on similar features with money allocated to nine districts on the basis of pre-set criteria, hospital reimbursement on the basis of diagnostic related groups and free choice of GPs and hospitals supported by GP advice. However, the decline of the county council-driven reforms such as the Dalarna and Stockholm models began during the centre-right government in early 1990s and thus centre-right governments, rather than social democrats, led the pull-backs from provider competition (Harrison and Calltorp 2000).

However, the centre-right government in Sweden did introduce more market-oriented polices opening up primary healthcare through the family doctors model. In the family doctors model money follows the patients on the basis of fee for service. However, it did not last long as it threatened the position and role of salaried doctors within primary healthcare (Twaddle 1999; Harrison and Calltorp 2000). The law also created the right to establish private practice in primary healthcare and enhanced competition between public and private sectors for the same resources. The law, initiated by the centre-right government, was weakened and effectively disbanded soon after the subsequent social democratic government came to power, while some county councils were allowed to continue with the model further. However, the centre-right government which gained power again in 2006 returned to the idea and in particular the issue of the right of establishment within an official report on patient rights (Socialdepartement 2007; SOU 2008a).

The reflection of municipal self-governance and the limits of decentralisation were felt in Sweden as county councils started contracting out services. This was also reflected in government work on steering health and social services in 1999 (SOU 1999a; 1999b). The best known example was St Görans hospital in Stockholm, which was politically important. Anticipating problems with future hospital sell offs in other counties, the social democratic government interfered and introduced the so-called 'stop-law' in 2001

(Regeringens Proposition 2004). The importance of the stop law is not only in the context of healthcare reform but also in relation to decentralisation and local autonomy. The centre-right government reversed this decision and repealed the law when it gained power in 2006 (Regeringens Proposition 2007).

The overall enthusiasm for healthcare reforms waned in the late 1990s as a result of escalation of medical costs and difficulties in governance alongside a general shift towards cooperation rather than competition (Harrison and Calltorp 2000; Whitehead *et al.* 1997; Harrison 2006). However, the later return of the conservative government in 2006 brought back many of the policies stalled by the social democratic government as well as initiated new policies with market-oriented features encouraging entrepreneurship in the health sector and enhancing patient choice in healthcare. The current debate remains still, however, strictly in the context of publicly financed services. The conclusions of the Ansvarskomitten (2007) – responsibility committee – that focused on the roles and responsibilities within the welfare state and in particular divisions between state and municipalities, in comparison to Norwegian centralisation measures, turned more towards information steering, gathering and provision of information in a way that resembles Finnish health system reforms 15 years ago.

Choice, patient rights and public participation

The competitive reforms at national level included different variations in the use of market mechanisms, contracting and related measures as well as the introduction of patient choice and care guarantees. These reforms were not based on law, but rather agreements between central government and county councils. The initial agreement on patient choice created choice of hospital for patients within the public services as well as a guarantee of care within a specified time limit. The scope of both of these measures was amended later in the 1990s.

According to Harrison and Calltorp, patient choice was popular with citizens and county council politicians, but only affected around 5 per cent of all patient visits between 1991 and 1993 and only 2–5 per cent of healthcare resources were reallocated as a result of the patient choice programme (Harrison and Calltorp 2000). However, in the context of the healthcare guarantee and patient choice, around 90 per cent of the patients who were offered an alternative in 1992 made a choice to wait a bit longer to get their treatment at their local hospital (Anell 1996).

The Swedish policy process is open to discussion and debate with extensive participation by experts and interested parties in the committee work. Policies are prepared by specific commissions and freedom of information legislation gives the public access to almost all official papers (Pollit and Bouckaert 2004). The issue of patient rights and public participation was clearly on the official agenda in the late 1980s and early 1990s even though Sweden never took the same legislative route as Finland in terms of patient rights. Furthermore, a large share of the 1980s reform measures promoting decentralisation and the healthcare reforms in the 1990s can now be seen as aiming to promote participation and 'democratic accountability'. A particular Swedish aspect of this reform agenda is the promotion of markets as a 'means' for furthering citizen choice and responsiveness (see Saltman 1986).

Ansvarskomitten (2007) proposed in its final report that a new patient law should cover patients' self-determination, choice and influence on care-decisions, patients' choice of longer term physician contact (e.g. GP, but not restricted to a GP and explicitly stated as right to choose a specialist), patient right to information on treatment and care, patient rights to compensation for damages and specific public bodies for patients and obligations for healthcare (Ansvarsnämden). In spite of the explicit tackling of patient's issues and widest ever consultation as part of the Committee report process, it is striking that the number of patient and other health organisations taking part in the consultation was very small.

Blomqvist (2004) has drawn attention to the nature and politics of promotion of choice in Swedish health policies. The role of patient choice has become even more important during the current centre-right government policies with engagement with government agencies such as the Competition Agency and Agency for Economic and Regional Growth (NUTEK) and private sector actors in the process of promoting choice. Government policies have concentrated on the broader choice context, where study visits have been made to Finland and Denmark. As a result the emphasis on 'permission to choose' covers not only healthcare, but a broad array of elderly care and social services (SOU 2008b). At the same time patient rights have become framed through the lens of choice. The government earlier in 1997 placed particular emphasis on patient rights (SOU 1997) with legislative measures addressing choice (Regeringens Proposition 1997; 1998).

The government's official report, while titled as one of patient rights in healthcare and how patients' position and influence could be strengthened, was not so much about patient rights as the right of establishment, which was presented as means to promote patient choice (Socialdepartementet 2007). The more detailed guidance provided scope to revisit the family doctor model, rights of establishment and patient choice (SOU 2008b). Patient rights were thus understood mostly in terms of the ability to exercise choice at the primary care level.

Patient choice has had a higher profile than patient rights in healthcare in Sweden. The new proposed mechanisms do little to shift this balance but rather raise questions about when equity in access or choice in rural areas will become more recognised. While there has been a general acceptance that patient choice reform has been well-liked and appreciated by citizens and municipal decision makers, this might overstate the importance of patient choice when set against other healthcare priorities. In this context the views of citizens seem to raise several other issues as higher priorities (Valentine *et al.* 2008).

The emergence on the political scene of the Health Service Party has an air of populist politics and it illustrates one of the ways in which health issues may be politicised in the context of local and national policy making (Sjukvårdspartiet 2008). On the other hand, it can also be seen as one of a number of single issue parties that emerge – and disappear – in the local policy arena. Another, more left-leaning, aspect of politicisation of health issues is the campaigning against the current commercialisation of welfare services through the 'network for our common welfare' (nätverk för gemensam välfärd). The network seems more Stockholm-centric with campaign against 'cream skimming' (gräddfil kampanj), although the capital is also where market policies have had the greatest impact and development (Nätverk för 2008).

Globalisation, European policies and national policy choices

In Sweden health policy development has been relatively insulated from European influences, which are recognised but remain marginal in most national debates. However, European policies have slowly emerged as salient, particularly in relation to reimbursement for the care costs. This is not the only case; there are other better known examples such as alcohol policies or pharmacy monopolies, which resulted in Sweden being taken to the European Court of Justice.

Health tourism or travelling to other countries in Europe for healthcare treatment, in the period 2004–2007 has remained concentrated primarily in dental care, which, together with two other disease groups, covered almost 80 per cent of those who sought care. Most trips were to Estonia, Finland, Germany, Spain and Poland. Of those patients who were reimbursed for planned care delivered elsewhere, 35 per cent went to Finland, while the largest costs were associated with highly specialised care delivered in Germany. In part the dominance of dental care can be explained by the fact that Sweden provides predominantly fixed sum reimbursement, whereas this is not the case for hospital care. The key factors promoting Swedish health tourism are waiting times or personal knowledge of another country. The number of patients, while these have risen, remained small in the context of the overall health system (Försäkringskassan 2007). As a result of European Union policies and national decisions Sweden also provides information on how to seek care outside the country. This results in patients often being more aware of how to access services in Estonia than in a neighbouring county council we were told.

Specific issues with respect to government procurement were identified in an official government report on procurement of health and social services in 1999 (SOU 1999a). Government procurement and competition requirements, including European legislation and court cases, were also considered in detail as part of the exploration for legislative proposals on user choice in local services (Konkurrensverket 2008; SOU 2008a). International examples in promoting user choice were, interestingly, raised in Finland as voucher schemes and in Denmark as part of the Government Competition Office work on enhancing competition in the area of health services (Viidas and Nilsson 2007). This report also emphasises that the principles established in the Treaty of the European Union should apply to the so-called Group B category services. These services, including health services, are not dealt with fully under the EU Directive on government procurement (ibid.) (see Chapter 6).

The broader implications of globalisation, it can be argued, are reflected through the articulation of business interests and their influence upon healthcare. The NUTEK[3] focus on the service sector and health and social services as a future commercial policy area reflects these interests by envisaging health services as a potential commercial growth area (NUTEK 2007a; 2007b). A joint publication of this government agency with the service industries association – Almega – considers health services as a sector with particular interest in patient focus and productivity (NUTEK and Almega 2007). This can also be seen as a form of 'opportunity'-driven globalisation as the main driver is not healthcare costs, which in Sweden have not been an issue since the 1990s, but the creation of health service industry as a *productive* sector of the economy.

The importance of European Union Working Time Directive was initially raised in Sweden through claims by local government of the necessity to employ 3000 new doctors to fill the gaps created through implementation (SKL 2004), a figure which was later disputed (Larsson *et al.* 2004). The issue has remained on the agenda of employer organisations including the Swedish Association of Local Authorities and Regions, with attention being drawn to the potential to use the opt-out from the directive as a welcome 'safety valve' (Bäckström *et al.* 2008).

The Ministry of Social Affairs and Health was, under the social democratic government, actively engaged with European policies and often took a critical stand towards proposed service directive and related provisions in the new proposed Constitutional Treaty. The new centre-right government on the other hand is actively pursuing other initiatives promoting patient choice and pluralism in service provision and considers health and social services a potential commercial sector. These seem to be less in conflict with European policies, for example, in relation to the application of patient rights in cross-border healthcare.

The politics and policies of public participation and commercialisation of care

Public participation and choice seem to have been at the core of the legitimacy and the initial impetus for health reform in Sweden; however, this emphasis

---

3 NUTEK (Swedish National Board for Industrial and Technical Development) was combined to form a part of a new agency Tillväxtverket, the Swedish Agency for Economic and Regional Growth on 01 April 2009 and also assumed the responsibilities of the Swedish National Rural Development Agency as well as the Swedish Consumer Agency's tasks concerning commercial and public services.

has given way to a more market-oriented understanding of the health system and consumer rather than patient needs. The emphasis on choice within Swedish health policies appears not to be driven by public expectation or practice but instead inspired by ideology among conservative politicians and free-market think tanks and personal interest among corporate and industrial employers; together they are the main drivers of these policies.

The general framework for service organisation was established in the context of broader decentralisation processes as part of broader public sector reform policies. As governments have changed over the last 20 years, conservative and centre-right governments have taken further steps towards commercialisation which social democratic governments have not reversed. This has created a fragmented, stuttering process of incremental policy change creating increased scope for further commercialisation.

The role of social democratic governments in accepting or promoting reform policies leading towards further commercialisation seems to be based essentially on the recognition of the focus on 'publicly financed' services. While reforms applying user charges have increased cost-sharing by users, the basic framework in Sweden has been predicated on publicly financed services. Currently service provision is relatively unregulated by government and based on cooperation through county councils. This also increases the importance of decentralisation for health policies. Decentralisation in itself implies that local elections count in defining service provision and obligations. This locus of power is reflected also in the context of reform policies and experiences, which vary across counties.

In Sweden there is a clear interest in the scope and potential of 'healthcare markets' as a future corporate growth area and thus an area of economic interest. This is reflected in the politics and assessment of the national health system. While the traditional problem area in the Swedish health system has been the relative weakness of primary healthcare in comparison to hospital-based care, this has been addressed only indirectly through the reform policies and proposals.

Health services and health systems issues appear to generate political interest in Sweden as reflected through the level of political activity and creation of specific health issue parties. However, at the same time ambitious policy proposals seem to slip through with little popular engagement or participation by nongovernmental organisations or patient groups.

The focus in Sweden on patients and participation is stronger on patient choice than on patient rights. The understanding of patients or service users as important in terms of involvement or participation in planning and developing services is not particularly strong. As patient focus seems to be driven to a large extent by those promoting choice and more entrepreneurial approaches to health services, other aspects of patient and public involvement do not seem to have gained substantial leverage. While Swedish policy making and practice of consultations is open to participation in general, the inclusion and engagement of users in planning services with some notable exceptions (Rosen 2006), is not as widely recognised. The challenge is that as democratic accountability for oversight over health services becomes distanced, there is a risk of over-reliance on patient choice as a steering mechanism for the benefit of patients within the system as a whole. Furthermore, there is a risk that in the politics of choice the choosing is increasingly done by providers rather than patients.

The role and relevance of the European Union to Swedish health services or local service provision has so far been limited. However, there is a longer standing national debate and focus on change in how market reforms have worked within the public sector as similar reforms have already been implemented in education (Dahlgren 1994; Blomqvist and Rothstein 2000). The idea of change and the necessity for change does not develop in a vacuum (see Blomqvist 2002; 2004; Blomqvist and Rothstein 2000), but the role of international actors, such as the OECD agencies has not been considered as an important influence on the Swedish policy process. Carrol (2004) suggests that Swedish decision makers have the capacity to resist OECD recommendations, to a greater or lesser degree depending on the politics of the current government, as domestic rather than exogenous forces present the most important political challenges.

The implications of globalisation seem to be channelled through three main pathways in Sweden. First, the impact of the economic crisis and initial concern over growing share of healthcare costs provided greater traction for economic arguments. Second, the diffusion of policy ideas – from new public management to the purchaser–provider split – reflect the role of globalisation in terms of the transmission of policy ideas. Third, the stronger voice of commercial and corporate actors and active policies to accommodate and promote entrepreneurship in the health system are apparent. Furthermore, the increasing engagement with the commercial sector in provision of healthcare makes the European Union internal markets framework more applicable to the Swedish health system. The challenge is then for the national policies to maintain both costs and solidarity within the publicly financed health system.

Conclusions

In Sweden patient and public participation in the health system has evolved in the context of policy reform through two routes, first that of democratisation and accountability with a focus on local level decentralisation, and second, in the context of patient choice.

The policy changes in health systems were initially supported by broad-based citizen dissatisfaction with health services. On the other hand enhancement of commercialisation and choice in healthcare can also be seen as part of a corporate sector agenda and the product of particular interest group activities. The articulation of patient choice has become intertwined with a discussion of a 'plurality' of providers that together legitimates the emergence of a revitalised private sector. The plurality of service providers is distinct from the earlier predominance of public services but remains distinct from privatisation because of continuing public financing. This shift in the environment is also apparent in Swedish corporate development as increasingly corporate actors are explicitly gearing their strategies towards public contracting markets.

While commercialisation has been initiated or implemented in order to promote participation, there remains a strong emphasis on democratic accountability as the basic mechanism for participation. At the same time the talk of empowering citizens and patients has been adopted by those promoting commercialisation. There is a danger that as service provision structures further separate from structures with electoral accountability, the expectations of democratic accountability as the basic form of participation will be challenged. Furthermore, the lack of direct public and patient involvement can and needs to be seen serving other needs in services development and culture.

Finally, in comparison to the potential vulnerability of the less-regulated Swedish health system to European Union policies and increasing emphasis on the four freedoms within Europe, Swedish policy making has remain separated from European policy developments. The reform policies in Sweden can be seen as an example of policy diffusion influenced by globalisation, although these were not identified as such during the reform process. The economic crisis further strengthened the market and economic policy arguments and the role of commercial and corporate interest groups within Swedish society and gave them added impetus in arguing for a change.

8   Finland
Commercialisation in the context of decentralised service provision

A shift in the relationship between citizen's rights, choice and commercialisation in Finland has taken place as part of broader policy changes. In this chapter we first analyse the context and background for policy changes, then focus on the actors involved in policy making and discuss the evolution of healthcare reform processes as well as citizens' and patients' rights and participation. We then focus on the relationship with international policies and conclude with our findings in relation to the Finnish case study.

The context and background for policy changes

The Finnish health system is a predominantly decentralised health system with a basic structure of publicly financed salaried health services provision complemented by National Health Insurance covering pharmaceutical reimbursement costs, partial reimbursement of private healthcare costs as well as for provision of occupational healthcare. Local governments are responsible for provision of health services with cross-subsidisation through state subsidies. The Finnish health system is predominantly tax-based and publicly funded through National Health Insurance (76 per cent in 2006), but complemented by cost-sharing by users (18.7 per cent in 2006) with the remaining share of funding from private insurance (2.2 per cent in 2006), non-profit institutions serving households (1.1 per cent in 2006) and employers (2 per cent in 2006) (STAKES 2008). For a more comprehensive description of the Finnish health system see Vuorenkoski (2008).

For more than a century Finnish local government municipalities have been responsible for providing basic health services. The number of municipalities has recently been reduced through mergers from 415 in 2004 to 348 from the beginning of 2009. During the 1950s and 1960s the majority of public expenditure on healthcare was allocated to hospitals and a significant imbalance between hospital care and outpatient care developed with particular limitations in primary healthcare. In 1972 a new system of primary healthcare was established through the Primary Health Care Act, which introduced municipal health centres as the basis of the primary care service. In the 1970s and 1980s increasing attention was placed on occupational health[4] services with the introduction of the Occupational Health Care Act in 1979 (Vuorenkoski 2008).

However, the Finnish health system retains some particular features that are a result of political compromises from when the health system was first founded. The National Health Insurance scheme was established in the 1960s to reimburse part of the costs of private healthcare. This, as well as the right of physicians to have private practice in addition to their salaried work, have remained a compromise from the initial model of the health system (see Keskimäki 2003; Vuorenkoski 2008). National Health Insurance provides reimbursement for a set part of costs for healthcare visits that take place in the private sector, pharmaceuticals, travel costs to health services, as well as reimburses part of the costs of occupational health services to the employer.

This initial structure is still reflected in the context of the two main resource channels – National Health Insurance and funding from municipal and central government – which have been a particular feature of the Finnish national health system (see Järvelin 2002; OECD 2005). The role of central government funding and guidance was important to the initial development of the health centre network and expansion of primary care services. Hospitals remain governed by one of the 20 hospital districts on mainland Finland while separate arrangements exist for the island of Åland (Vuorenkoski 2008).

The governance of municipal services is based on elected municipal councils who appoint the members of municipal health boards. The locally elected representatives have an indirect governance role in health services through these arrangements. Municipalities share the power to appoint members of the hospital councils as the main governance arrangements in hospital districts. The council approves membership of hospital executive boards that direct the practical administration of the hospital.

Reforms of municipal services were initiated in the 1970s, but were only implemented in the 1980s. The Valtava reform changed the planning process and the ways in which state subsidies were allocated preceded this with preparatory work taking place in the mid 1970s (Niemelä 2008). These reforms essentially shifted the agenda from expansion to maintenance. Through the late 1980s and 1990s public sector reforms in the planning, steering and financing of public services were mostly inspired by New Public Management concepts.

---

4 In the Finnish context Occupational Healthcare covers primary healthcare of the working population. Employers are obliged to provide their employees with preventive healthcare, and may if they wish, also arrange medical treatment and other health services. The Social Insurance Institution reimburses the employer for 50 per cent of all necessary and reasonable costs incurred in providing occupational healthcare, while the municipal health centre must be prepared to arrange occupational health services to those employers who want to acquire them (STM 2004).

There were three key changes framed by New Public Management-inspired reforms. First, in the name of municipal and local autonomy, earmarked funds previously allocated to municipal health services were now allocated on the basis of a given profile of healthcare needs and area specific characteristics. This change was further developed as part of the Social and Health Services Planning and State Subsidy Act (1992). Second, alongside the right to decide how services are provided came in the financial responsibility for these decisions, accompanied by the establishment of a municipality's right to charge healthcare users. This new principle was established through the User-Fees in Social and Health Care Act (1992) and was mainly intended to eliminate 'unnecessary healthcare visits', rather than the promotion of self-sustained funding. Third, the economic crisis in the early 1990s initiated a broader shift in thinking about public services with a greater focus on productivity and efficiency in the context of the necessity to cut public sector costs of which health and social services cover substantial part in municipalities.

An emphasis on democratic accountability inspired efforts to promote municipal self-governance. The initial moves were based on pressures for decentralisation and municipal self-governance but formed in practice a legal framework of rights and responsibilities for health and social services. In principle the separation of purchaser and provider responsibilities was established through this process, however, its implementation remained limited throughout the 1990s. The role of direct central government funding of health expenditure has declined from over 36 per cent in 1990 to 23 per cent in 2006 (STAKES 2007; 2008). The overall financing continues to depend on multiple funding channels (see Table 8.1). The economic crisis in Finland created a new context for healthcare reforms that increasingly emphasised scarcity and improving the efficiency of service provision. These aims were accompanied by the broader implementation of public sector reforms in the early 1990s.

Table 8.1 Health expenditure by source of funding 1995–2006

	1995	2000	2005	2006
General government	74.1	73.4	75	76
General government except social security funds	61.3	59.1	60	61.1
Central government	27.2	18.4	21.9	22.6
Local government	34.0	40.7	38.1	38.5
Social security funds	12.8	14.3	15	14.9
Private sector	25.9	26.6	25	24
Private social insurance	0.5	0.5	0.4	0.4
Private health insurance	2.0	2.1	1.8	1.8
Out-of-pocket payments	20.5	21	19.6	18.7
Non-profit institutions serving households	1.2	1.1	1.2	1.1
Employers and corporations	1.7	1.9	2.0	2.0

Source: STAKES: Health expenditure and financing (2007; 2008).

In terms of the organisation and steering of the Finnish health system, the focus on municipal autonomy with centrally set obligations relying increasingly on locally collected funds has been problematic. The population base in many localities is small and the capacity for municipalities to govern hospital costs are limited, resulting in a greater focus on cost-savings potential within municipal health and social services. While there was cross-subsidisation through central funding, it is clear that particularly smaller municipalities encountered difficulties when presented with patients needing costly treatment, such as cancer care.

Specific recentralisation measures were taken in relation to particular services leading to central government intervention in the field of child psychiatric services in order to ensure that resources were used for this purpose (STM 2001). The overall sense of economic stringency and lack of resources dominated policies and were further exacerbated at the end of 1990s by strike action by medical doctors.

In the late 1990s a new emphasis on healthcare was initiated by the national government. The preparatory process led to a government resolution in 2002 on securing the future of healthcare focusing on, amongst other issues, strengthening primary healthcare and addressing issues of access and financing of healthcare. The implementation using tightly defined projects limited the impact of these changes (STM 2002; STM 2008a). In relation to health services and citizen's rights, the main consequence of this process was the 'care guarantee'. While not necessarily considered part of patient rights, the regulation of 'care guarantee' through national legislative act for access to treatment in non-urgent specialised care was initiated in early 2000 and enacted in 2005 (Valtioneuvoston asetus 2005). These actions were aimed at shortening queues, but also reflected a perceived need to strengthen the universal basis for access as part of the efforts rather than leaving this to the vagaries of local municipal governments. The 'care guarantee' can also be seen as a return to a more normative regulatory approach. In addition to the legislation on the 'care guarantee', the implementation was largely through project funding and was also relatively ineffective.

Citizen's rights and patient rights

In terms of citizen's rights, two major developments were initiated during the 1990s. First, the legislation on patient rights, the Status and Rights of Patients Act came into force in 1993 and focused on how and what patients could expect from health service providers, including the establishment of an ombudsman in each healthcare unit. The Act was established after a long preparatory phase and on the basis of our interviews international social rights and the European Social Charter provided the context and legislative framework for the Act.

The revision of the Finnish Constitution came into force in March 2000 and set out the rights to access healthcare through obligating public authorities to guarantee adequate social, health and medical services for all residents and promote the health of the population (Finnish Constitution 1999). However, two issues are important in this context: first, constitutional rights do not obligate public authorities to provide, but merely to guarantee services. Second, alongside the patient rights legislation, these Constitutional rights are based on residence.

Complaints where treatment has led to death or severe injury of the patients are normally dealt with by the National Authority for Medico-legal Affairs (NAMLA) (Vuorenkoski 2008). In 2006 the role of NAMLA was widened to cover health services and in January 2009 it was combined with The National Product Control Agency for Welfare and Health (STTV) to form the National Supervisory Authority for Welfare and Health (Valvira) (Valvira 2009a). The number of complaints has risen each year and those made by patients and relatives have risen from around 200 in the early 2000s to slightly above 300 per year during 2007–2009 (Valvira 2009b).

Consumer rights legislation applies solely to private services and their purchase. The use of purchasing for publicly financed services has created concern and a lack of clarity regarding the responsibilities with respect to services purchased by local municipal governments. However, the responsibility for purchased services remains with the local government even if the services are provided by a private sector organisation. The consumer authority has drawn attention to this issue and has emphasised that the division of responsibilities between the producer and contractor are clear and that consideration is paid to ensuring availability and continuity of services (Consumer Agency 2006).

In theory the members of the population have the possibility to choose between municipal health services, private health services and occupational health services with additional health services available for students. On the other hand, this choice is affected by the user charges in primary health services and private health services as the National Health Insurance only partially reimburses private sector fees. Furthermore, private services are mostly available in urban areas. Occupational health services are available only to employed persons; such services are free for the employee and create a priority channel for accessing services for those who are employed. For employees services are only available from the provider chosen by the employer and include only those services and investigations that have been agreed.

The report on the position of the customer in 1998 by the Ministry of Social Affairs and Health concluded that, comparatively, the position for Finnish users of the health services was generally good. The culture of participation, however, is not very strong, and the role of consumer and patient associations remains rather limited. Further, there is little opportunity for patients to choose either a doctor or the location or timing of an appointment (STM 1998). In a survey of patients in 1997 respondents considered the most important issue was the ability to receive treatment when needed and to be treated well, to be provided with sufficient information relating to individual health status and treatment alternatives; choice however was ranked 12 out of 17 in importance (Pekurinen *et al.* 1997).

Commercialisation and health service provision

Nongovernmental actors have been involved in the Finnish healthcare system in three types of activity. First, nongovernmental organisations were involved in service provision, including the establishment of hospitals. Second, the establishment and presence of traditional for-profit corporate sector actors until the 1990s were primarily group practices of doctors. Third, the establishment of new models of service trading activity, such as medical services firms and the replacement of physician employment relationships to personal service contracts, allowed the application of arrangements possible for corporations, including lower corporate taxes, rather than more progressive income tax.

The key legislative changes enabling the commercialisation and contracting out of services and increased cost-sharing by users were initially implemented in the late 1980s and 1990s. While the scope for contracting out in municipalities was created early on, the lack of resources and capacity limited the formal outsourcing of municipal services. Furthermore, the lack of market mechanisms in municipal services made outsourcing more difficult in practice. The National Slot-Machine Association can be understood as an additional resource channel. The National Slot-Machine Association was established in 1938 to raise funds through gaming operations to support Finnish health and welfare organisations.

On the other hand, the expansion of occupational health services has created an opportunity for private sector providers. A substantial number of larger employers, including government institutions, provide occupational health services to their employees through contractual arrangements with private sector providers. This approach has been supported by the government for preventive and curative services.

However, in terms of commercialisation, the 1990s were dominated by the promotion of markets and competition by other government actors, initiated, in particular, by the Office for Competition. The Office for Competition reacted to the 'monopoly' in the public sector in the late 1990s by questioning the 'monopoly' supplier status of public services (Kilpailuvirasto 1996; 2001). However, in the 1990s the promotion of competition and market mechanisms was more oriented towards the public sector rather than to engaging with private providers and markets. The engagement with private actors has become more prominent during the last ten years.

The promotion of market mechanisms, such as vouchers and contracting from private sector providers, long remained marginalised to pilot studies and specific projects (Lith 2001; 2006). Incrementally, market mechanisms are more broadly promoted and practised by the Ministry of Trade and Industry. Since 2000, and particularly since the change in government in 2007, contracting with the private sector has had a higher profile within the Ministry of Social Affairs and Health. This is also reflected in the promotion of vouchers and patient choice in health services, as well as levelling the ground between private and public provision in terms of, for example, price, VAT regulations, and the possibility to use public premises for private provision.

The role of markets has increased through four processes. First, the fact that medical doctors have been allowed to maintain private, but publicly subsidised, practice and to do this in addition to their public sector work provides an established presence and basis for the expansion by private providers. Second, the role of private practice in occupational health services provided a predictable and steady basis for service development. Third, the introduction of user charges and problems of staff recruitment in the public sector have shifted public perception of the service. User charges have diminished the difference between public and private sector and professional staff shortages have created the scope for commercialisation of professional services but with higher costs. This has also been affected by the earlier commercialisation of more informal practices in securing night-time and weekend practices. Fourth, additional measures are creating greater demand for private sector in the context of care guarantee and the removal of the so-called 'band-aid tax', which changed the agreement to treat accidents and injuries of insured patients in the public sector and opened these 'markets' to the private sector (Valtioneuvoston asetus 2004; Mehiläinen 2005; Kilpailuvirasto 2006).

The role of private health insurance has been of greater importance with respect to children, accidents and injuries, which have often been included as part of travel or home insurance. It has been estimated that in 2005, 375,000 children and 237,000 adults had voluntary private health insurance, while about one fifth of the population had leisure time and sporting accident insurance in 2005 (Vuorenkoski 2008).

Until the 1990s these private health services were primarily professional group practices owned by professionals rather than commercially driven services. During the 1990s the structure of private providers and their orientation had changed with both international ownership and more commercially oriented professional management and leadership of the organisations. Medical group practices have become dominated by chains with the two main national chains providing private sector medical and occupational health services (Terveystalo and Mehiläinen). Mehiläinen joined Swedish Carema in 2006 as both were bought by H-Careholding, which changed its name to Ambea AB in 2007. It is owned by a British private equity company 3i and GIC, an investment management company owned by the Singapore Government (Mehiläinen 2008). Terveystalo was mostly Finnish owned with a substantial stake held by the Mutual Pension Insurance Companies and reportedly only 1 per cent foreign ownership in 2008 (Terveystalo 2008).[5]

5 In 2009 Terveystalo was bought by a new company, Star Healthcare Oy, established by Bridgepoint Capital Ltd.

However, the number of acquisitions made by Terveystalo during recent years implies that competition within the corporate sector is likely to become more of an issue. The idea of empowered individual consumers making choices from a variety of competing providers seems unlikely, but rather the emergence of corporate monopoly provision, particularly in the light of the larger contracting potential created by the municipal services reform, would seem more likely.

The role of private hospitals has become more prominent in areas where demand can be created (e.g. laser surgery, plastic surgery). The role of private hospitals has also evolved in the context of charitable and church-related work (e.g. Diacor-hospital) and a specific focus on particular diseases often with nongovernmental organisations active in these spheres (e.g. Reuman-hospital and the Orton-hospital). The margin between for-profit and not-for-profit actors is not always clear and it is likely that the more competitive and commercially oriented the sector becomes, the more it will shape and influence the ways in which these actors can and will engage with service provision.

The magnitude of contracting out is also likely to be larger than shown in official statistics as some aspects of contracting, such as the hiring of doctors, do not appear in statistics (Fredriksson and Martikainen 2006; Lith 2006). The current estimates of the magnitude of private sector involvement indicate that private sector providers in health and social care accounted for 23 per cent of all costs of services and covered 20 per cent of personnel in 2003 (Kauppinen and Niskanen 2005).

The actors and institutional context in Finnish health policies

Finnish health policy actors are similar to those in other countries in terms of the role and relevance of medical doctors and nurses as professional groups. However, municipalities are an additional actor within the policy-making community because of their responsibilities for provision. The role of nongovernmental organisations has been important in promoting public health policies but many organisations have also been involved with service provision. Their role has been more limited in terms of influencing health systems and structures within health systems beyond their own service provision efforts and most disease- or condition-based groups focus on substantive issues in health policies and health promotion efforts. While our interviews indicate that there have been some efforts to engage different groups, these have been mostly related to projects rather than systematic efforts to participate.

In health policies the role of professional organisations and trade union activity has been prominent, including strikes by both medical doctors in 2001 on pay and working conditions and nurses in 2007 on pay. Professional organisations, such as the Duodecim Society, have traditionally been involved in more substantive matters.

Decentralisation of service provision results in major policies being developed in relation to municipalities. While the Finnish Association of

Municipalities does not carry as much weight as the Association of Swedish County Councils, it could be argued that it is seeking a clearer role in the area.

Private sector providers have become more engaged with the policy process and issues, however, the promotion of commercialisation is more clearly mediated through engagement with the Ministry of Trade and Industry, Ministry of Finance, think tanks and employer and business interest organisations and institutes. The role of the Ministry of Trade and Industry in this field has been proactive. It has also focused on new areas of engagement by seeking to commercialise public health and social services as part of export promotion efforts (Kauppa ja-teollisuusministeriö 2007). This is reflected in the views that health services have underdeveloped export potential and there is a necessity to open public services to private competition so as to enhance development of health services as a more viable export sector. The efforts of the driving forces within the Ministry of Trade and Industry could be best understood in the context of promoting commercial policies, export potential and productivity. The concern in this respect is that development and regulation is no longer primarily driven by health or citizen concerns, but on the basis of the prospects for the sector to provide the basis for commercial development.

The role of trade unions is important in the context of the overall corporatist history of national policies and has also influenced the development and practice of occupational health service provision. Thus far there have been few prominent public local campaigns around particular hospitals with the exception of the historical mental health hospital in Lapinlahti and the maternity department of Tammisaari local hospital. National health policies changed in the 1990s due to decentralisation and emphasis on information steering. While institutions, such as the National Research and Development Centre for Social Welfare and Health (STAKES), have provided comprehensive information resources, the tightening economic resource base within municipalities has had consequences for their ability to develop and implement effective policies. Institutional support to municipalities was also given through other mechanisms; the Ministry of Trade and Industry provides advice on government procurement as well as channelling funds through the TEKES programme on health technology development. A new TEKES programme has also been initiated jointly with the Ministry of Social Affairs and Health on innovations in health service provision, including, in particular, customer-driven approaches (TEKES 2008).

The role of industry and demands of corporate actors have been channelled through think tanks, employers and corporate associations and individual companies and their representatives. This is apparent in the work of these actors on broader welfare state issues but also exerts an influence in relation to particular health or health related issues. Health has been taken up in the context of the work of the Research Institute of the Finnish Economy (ETLA) and Finnish Business and Policy Forum (EVA) (see Rouvinen *et al.* 1995; Kanniainen 2002). The Finnish Chamber of Commerce has, for example, presented a model for care vouchers (Kauppakamari 2008). The Finnish Innovation Fund (SITRA) has a dual role as a funder and as a think tank. As a think tank it has been actively involved in healthcare issues and emphasise the need to change the context of national policy making. Its dual role gives a broader impact based on connections to investors in the area and the capacity to utilise close links with policy makers, which could be seen also as a conflict of interests in terms of health policies. The relationship between SITRA, TEKES and Ministry of Trade and Industry is close, with a greater distance between them and the more health and social policy focused institutions including STAKES and the National Health and Social Insurance Institution (KELA) and the Ministry of Social Affairs and Health.

Healthcare reform as part of public sector reform

The major healthcare reforms have been part of broader municipal and public service reforms. The initial strengthening of primary healthcare in the context of the establishment of the national health system in the 1970s and early 1980s shifted to focus on hospital care in the 1990s. In Finland commercialisation has not been linked to the 'empowerment' of primary healthcare or other measures to strengthen the role of primary healthcare. A particular feature has been the declining role of public health measures and the diminishing health presence within schools, while at the same time occupational health services have expanded incrementally. In many ways the developments that have taken place in the commercialisation of Finnish primary healthcare conflict with aims for more comprehensive public health and prevention-oriented primary healthcare.

The increasing role of local governments in financing services has contributed to this change. The reasons for the relatively stronger squeeze on public health measures and primary healthcare services can at least partially be explained by the simple fact that the reimbursement of hospital costs are relatively inflexible to local pressure leaving resource savings to be found mainly from locally provided services and preventive health activities. This is also why the integration of social and health services is more problematic at the local municipality level.

Healthcare reform policies were embedded in the context of broader public sector reform with the aim to separate providers and purchasers and enhance contracting out of services. The framework and possibilities for this were set in the State Subsidies Act in 1992. A longer period of shifts in municipal self-governance and decentralisation were on the agenda during the 1980s creating the basis for the State Subsidies Act. These reforms were also actively promoted by business proponents (Finnish Business and Policy Forum, EVA) and more conservative policy makers. The public sector reform efforts in relation to private service providers were part of the conservative-centre party Holkeri government programme in 1987 (see Table 8.2). These reforms were presented in the context of improving services and

142   *Finland*

Table 8.2 National governments 1987–2007

Duration	Prime Minister	Party	Position
1987–1991	Holkeri	National coalition (Conservatives)	right-centre
1991–1995	Aho	Centre party	centre-right
1995–2003	Lipponen	Social-democrat	left-right
2003–2007	Vanhanen	Centre party	centre-left
2007–	Vanhanen	Centre party	centre-right

strengthening the self-governance of municipalities, which became even stronger during the subsequent Aho centre-conservative government (Forma *et al.* 2007a).

Thus, the Valtava reforms that allowed municipalities to purchase services from the private sector can be seen as part of this broader process. However, there was no privatisation of health services during the 1980s and since 1975 there have been no major changes in terms of finances, users or the distinction between private and public sector (Häkkinen 1987). On the other hand, the context for these activities changed during the late 1980s and 1990s as government subsidies declined and municipalities were left with legal obligations but declining resources. While market mechanisms and corporate sector actors were presented primarily as a means to promote efficiency, the actual use of markets and competitive mechanisms has been limited in health and social services. In the early 2000s some municipalities developed cooperative arrangements with other municipalities or entered into enhanced cooperation with for-profit or non-profit providers. The role of actual purchaser–provider arrangements in provision of services has been more limited and four out of five municipal social directors considered that it has little or no role in social and health services (Eronen *et al.* 2006). Thus, while municipalities have been given rights to decide on what basis they provide services in health services this has not led to substantial corporate sector engagement.

One important context for decision making in this area has been the public procurement regulations. The Finnish procurement law originates from Finland joining the EEA, the European Economic Area, in 1994 as it was obliged to change local legislation to comply with European Union government procurement directives. In the early 1990s the Ministry of Trade and Industry prepared national legislation that in effect went further than the European Union directive in terms of coverage and minimum requirements. The legislation was in essence based on the Ministry's orientation to enhance competition and increase public sector efficiency. Initially the view of the Ministry of Social Affairs and Health was that it would be rare for procurement under this directive to be utilised (Romppainen 2003). Romppainen goes on to argue that the policy process led by the Ministry of Trade and Industry was still driven on the basis of principles of inclusion, even though it was not assumed to be of relevance to social and health services.

There are clear interests in using public procurement policies to enhance the role of the private sector in contractual markets. Since 2005 the Finnish Chamber of Commerce has had its own project aiming to develop public procurement markets, increase the role of firms in the provision of public services and support, cooperation between firms and public procurement units with the aim that service providers are chosen in ways that respect the principles of a market economy (Kauppakamari 2008).

The promotion of the purchaser–provider split, competition and commercialisation of health services need to be understood as a trade and industry driven strategy. The Ministry of Trade and Industry has consistently promoted outsourcing of services as well as different types of voucher schemes (see Kauppa-ja teollisuusministeriö 2001). These aims have been articulated explicitly in the context of concerns over future demographic change, globalisation and productivity with core of the policy articulation taking place outside the Ministry of Social Affairs and Health framed by broader service reform until the change of government in 2007. It is in this context that the latest phase of the national project on modernisation of services structures takes place.

While the national project was initiated by the Vanhanen centre-left government, the process has continued with a two-fold structural emphasis during the Vanhanen centre-right government (Vanhanen 2004). The government proposal aims to, first, create forms of provision that are sufficiently large and more easily amenable to outsourcing through competitive mechanisms. Second, assumptions relating to a population base of 20,000 are substantially larger than the average size of Finnish municipalities. This implies that the municipalities need to reform their service-provision substantially, whether through mergers, cooperation or other arrangements. Therefore in many municipalities the direct political accountability for services provision and the financing of services may become separated. However, while the proposed framework law sets conditions for further commercialisation and change in provision of care, it does not exclude the provision of services as joint services.

In 2007 Parliament adopted the Municipal and Service System Reform Act, that is the framework law for reform of municipal service provision. The population basis for social and health service provision is 20,000. It has been estimated that this would require around 70 cooperative regions within the country (Kuntaliitto 2008). While this process takes service provision out of the direct oversight of those municipalities that have less than 20,000 inhabitants, it remains unclear whether and how oversight under the new model will be organised. In particular, it is unclear what scope will exist for the inclusion of the views of services users during the planning and implementation phases. The role of users or participation in this context has gained little attention. Niemelä (2008) has pointed out that in the light of earlier arguments on democracy and self-governance the focus at the end of 1990s on local government structures was based on a different emphasis. The arguments relating to democracy and local self-governance were almost totally absent and in contrast the aim was to enhance productivity and cost-efficiency through appropriate mergers. The focus on diminishing resources and the challenges of financing local services has remained an important part of national health policies, although later arguments have emphasised the impact of an aging population, globalisation or aspects of productivity.

From patient rights to consumer choice

The establishment of the patient rights legislation, Status and Rights of Patients Act 1993, was the result of a ten-year process. The underlying drivers for this process have been obligations arising from the European Social Charter rather than particular pressure from patient and interests groups. The Finnish law on patient rights was first to emerge in Europe, a year prior to the equivalent Act in the Netherlands (Partanen and Martikainen 1994; Sheldon 1994). The Act has been challenging to implement, particularly in terms of the establishment in all healthcare units of patient ombudsmen to help patients with information sharing and complaints.

A national review of patient ombudsmen found several problems with respect to the system and its functioning. In particular they found a lack of attention to conflicts of interest arising from ombudsmen being staff in the same unit where they should be promoting patient rights (Aho 2004). An initiative to amend the law was made in parliament in 2006 (Sirnö 2006). Fallberg (2000) has criticised the Finnish law as being labelled a 'law of rights', but built on obligations of staff and healthcare organisations to the patient; the right to care in this context is not an absolute legal right as it is limited by resources on the basis of the first article of the Act. He also suggests that regulations regarding patients' consent to care and treatment are absent implying an assumption of 'silent' or 'presumed' consent. On the other hand, the weaknesses in the ombudsmen system could be addressed, but taking up the issue in the national health system would require political will. Ensuring that the ombudsmen system functions meaningfully in the context of expanded patient choice and new providers entering the market is a challenge.

The national constitutional law is important in terms of ensuring rights to access healthcare for residents within municipalities as well as obligations on local governments to organise these services. While the government is obliged to ensure that all citizens have access to care, this need not be ensured through public services or that public services should be provided universally, as long as the government takes care that universal services are provided (Oikeus ja Kohtuus 2006). The United Kingdom Citizen's Charters have also found their way to Finland. However, the context and application of citizen charters in social and health services has become focused on quality-related technical aspects, with an emphasis on provider and local government transparency of what citizens may expect from the services (Haverinen 1999).

Choice of health services in Finland in practice is quite limited. While people are legally entitled to choose, when possible, the hospital specialist, this is not necessarily broadly recognised. Choice has mainly functioned to provide access to a second opinion and as an opt-out to the private sector rather than as primary consumer choice. Choice is even more limited in primary health-care where people have had to attend the health centre assigned to them, with varying opportunities to choose a particular doctor in that one health centre.

During the second Lipponen and first Vanhanen governments, studies on the prospects and use of vouchers were conducted. The first regulations concerning vouchers in social and health services were developed in 2004 when vouchers could be used for home care. This was extended to home nursing in 2008. Amendments to the legislation are being proposed to extend the use of vouchers more broadly across social and health services (STM 2008b). The proposed healthcare law also engages with the choice agenda setting it in the context of choice within public services and broadening it to include hospital services (STM 2008c). The promotion of choice has been driven by the assumed benefits from consumer choice and the importance of creating pluralism (i.e. choices) in service provision. However, in practice this is limited by the majority of private providers being concentrated in urban areas and in southern Finland.

The tradition of providing patient information or guidance for services is not strong in Finland. Considering the conceptualisation of Finland as a high-tech society, there is relatively little formal guidance on services provided by the public sector to inform citizens. These activities have become the domain of nongovernmental organisations, professional associations and also to some extent the pharmaceutical industry that has supported the development and production of some patient materials under the auspices of patient organisations.

Population-based surveys have not found particular support for individual private sector services but rather demonstrate support for a more public service-based approach. A 2006 survey by Forma concluded that:

> The results reveal strong support for the current welfare state system. The majority of the respondents were not willing to cut social spending even if such cuts would be accompanied by tax reductions. Similarly, the majority of the respondents would be willing to pay more taxes if the increased tax revenues were earmarked to health expenditures, pensions or child benefits.
>
> (Forma *et al.* 2007b: 52)

Another analysis of results from surveys of population views on the commercialisation of municipal services in 1996, 2000 and 2004 concluded that ideology and local political constituencies explained best the views presented. The results also demonstrated that support for the commercialisation of services has diminished and differences in attitudes have grown between 1996 and 2004. Alongside the change in services a change in citizens' views has followed in a more critical direction of change (Kallio 2007). These findings totally conflict with the policies promoted by successive governments in the name of citizen demands. The support for welfare state and public services is also reflected in the surveys overseen by EVA, the Finnish Business and Policy Forum. The EVA survey in 2007 found continuous support for solidarity, the welfare state and a lack of support for the privatisation or contracting out of public services (Haavisto *et al.* 2007).

Globalisation, European policies and national health policy choices

The impact of globalisation and European policies in Finnish health policy choices is mediated through three avenues: the impact of new public management approaches, considering health services as a tradable commodity and the expansion of legal and regulatory constraints.

1   Narrowing financial policy space: the emphases on downsizing the public sector, as an international political trend, expressed in, for example, part of new public management and the economic criteria adopted by the EU and the EMU. Together with the impact of the Finnish economic crisis in the early 1990s the emphasis on reducing the share of public resources that are spent in the health sector, has strengthened the economic and cost-containment arguments. While the share of public funding for social and health services remains low in relation to international standards (Heikkilä *et al.* 2007), an emphasis in policy debates on productivity and effectiveness within the health and social sectors has emerged as a dominant theme.

2   Changing values and priorities to conceptualise health as a commercial sector: the dominance of the Ministries of Trade and Industry and Finance in policy making has led to an emphasis on productivity, competitiveness and innovation. This shift is understandable as the role of traditional industrial sectors in the Finnish economy decline in importance. These shifts, together with the realisation that health services could be considered a rapidly growing business sector internationally has made the industrial and trade perspective more dominant for framing health services. While the role of the economic and commercial policy ministries has traditionally been stronger in comparison to the Ministry of Social Affairs and Health, the priorities of other ministries now extend further and more deeply into the national health policy space. This change is also influenced in part by the implementation of new public management policies and guidance from international organisations such as the OECD.

3   The expanding legal and regulatory context narrows the policy space for health. The context within which Finnish health policies are developed

and implemented has changed. The role and content of European Union health policies has altered and the impact of internal market regulation has also impacted other European countries. The impact of global trade agreements remains limited in Finland, although formal aspects of the internal market regulatory measures such as multilateral, plurilateral and bilateral trade agreements have similarities with global regulatory measures.

Finnish municipalities have historically been important and relatively autonomous actors. However, in national health policies decentralisation has enabled commercialisation through three avenues: first, the weakening of power and more limited voice in articulating policy priorities at a national level. Second, the mixed obligations and potential for blame shifting between central and local governments. Third, the lack of capacity, oversight and power in municipalities to follow and respond to changes promoted within other sectors, in particular, if these are implemented as national or European Union requirements. While the Ministry of Social Affairs and Health is usually considered a weaker ministry, the process of decentralisation may have further weakened its position to articulate national policy issues and generate significant allies.

The traditional comparison and context for policy change in Finland has been with the other Nordic countries, particularly Sweden. The experience of other Nordic countries is usually part of the way that new legislative proposals are contextualised. The role of Great Britain has also been important due to the more accessible language, but in the 1990s study expeditions to the United States were also undertaken by a range of policy actors.

The role of international organisations has been important in shaping health policy, with the WHO and ILO from 1950s through 1970s influencing health and social policies and occupational health and safety. However, in the 1980s the role of public policies in general and public sector reform policies in particular brought more attention to the OECD. In our interviews with civil servants in the Ministry of Social Affairs and Health, the WHO and OECD were mentioned in the context of international comparisons and their relevance to national policy making. The role of the OECD has also been important in promoting new public management reforms often through published reviews of the Finnish healthcare system. However, some of the initial focus on competition was also associated with OECD work on competition and regulatory reform.

In European policies the initial national policy stance was to ignore the EU in relation to health services because of subsidiarity as it had been assumed that joining the European Union would not affect the provision of health services. The role and relevance of European policies has slowly become of greater interest but has been debated more openly in the context of government procurement and the Finnish stance with respect to the proposed EU Constitutional Treaty.

In the case of active European health policies, the Ministry of Social Affairs and Health proposed that Treaty provision measures would allow shared competence and an exception from majority voting in trade negotiations in the area of health and social services. Further, that health services would be considered an exception from internal market rules. In the light of the discussions and developments concerning legal certainty this position could have provided explicit and substantial certainty in relation to internal markets (see Chapter 5). The exclusion of health from internal markets did not, however, gain sufficient support but instead the trade-related emphasis gained greater national and international support with the result that support was given to a narrow 'emergency break' option initially proposed by Sweden. The difficulty in the process was not merely having a national stance on the principle, but also gaining adequate support from those involved in the actual negotiations. This was complicated by the recognition that what were being presented were 'defensive' measures and against ordinary policy position, and thus potentially problematic to negotiators more committed to strengthening EU effectiveness and the success of the Treaty. The lack of understanding of the problem for national policy priorities was remedied at least in part by joint action from the Ministries of Social Affairs and Health and Education with broader popular activism helping to highlight the cause.

In terms of globalisation, Europe and national policy processes the politics and process in relation to the European Constitutional Treaty is interesting as it underscored the importance of public participation and parliamentary accountability for decisions where inter-ministerial exchanges are unlikely to be successful. Furthermore, it provided an example of the importance of European cooperation on European health policy issues.

The issue of internal markets and health was again debated in the context of the proposal on the services directive, but after initial changes to accommodate the concerns of the Ministry of Social Affairs and Health, the Finnish national policy stance was withdrawn and became integrated into the position of the Ministry of Trade and Industry in favour of including health services as part of the directive. The change in policy emphasis in the Ministry of Social Affairs and Health is hard to explain on the basis of resolved issues (e.g. country of origin) in the negotiation process, but seem to be instead a result of the changes in power positions and strengthening of the role of Ministry of Trade and Industry in this field, as the actor responsible for national policy coordination on the matter. On the other hand, the process also reflects the problematic context of 'joint' decision making across ministries.

The politics and policies of public participation and commercialisation of care

Public support and legitimacy for policy measures can be generated 1) by responding to expressed demands from patients and the public in the form of political campaigning (voice), and 2) in responding to priorities expressed in the context of, for instance, surveys of the views of citizens. In Finland the enhancement of commercialisation and choice seems to fail in relation to both accounts.

The politics of competition within the public sector, patient choice and increasing plurality in services provision (i.e. engagement of the private sector either in the form of NGOs or for-profit agencies) needs to be seen more as a political priority driven by other aims in Finland. The explicit *technical aims* of the Office of Competition, Ministry of Trade and Industry and Ministry of Finance are clear and supported by national corporate think tanks, such as EVA and the 'parliamentary' think tank SITRA, whose funds are heavily invested in the healthcare industry. In this articulation competition is a means to promote effectiveness and choice a mechanism for responding to users.

The Finnish Medical Association has been positively oriented towards promoting competition and choice in healthcare and has also engaged in direct discussions with the Ministry of Trade and Industry. On the basis of policy documents, the Finnish Medical Association has been supportive of patient choice, but also the role of public financing (Saarinen 2007a). However, the stance of medical doctors as such seems to be less embracing of markets, with a more critical stance towards commercialisation where this has taken place (Saarinen 2007b). The national association and trade union of nurses has remained less interested in competition and cost-containment, as reflected, for example, in policy issues raised by the union in the 2008 municipal elections (TEHY 2008). The trade union for municipal workers and public sector employees has also remained critical towards commercialisation. However, it is clear, that their voice has not been very strong in the context of overall changes within municipal services. The association of municipalities has traditionally had an office in Brussels to follow up European policies. However, the interests and emphases of the municipalities and their representatives are also framed in the context of the broader impact of European policies upon the availability and nature of national subsidies, the framing of public service provision and the scope for support for economic development.

The national umbrella organisation for social and health NGOs also compiled a document on internal markets and health and social services during the Finnish EU presidency (Palola 2007). However, the focus of NGO campaigning has remained primarily on issues particular to their interests, such as the role and definition of services of general interests.

Considering that there is no active pursuit of commercialisation of health services, patient choice or increasing access to private sector health services by a range of key stakeholders, the pressure for these forms of policy solutions more likely a result of commercial provider or professional organisation lobbying or the product of ideologically driven politics. It is clear that the existing private sector providers and doctors have argued for choice and are likely to argue for more generous social insurance support to enable this. However, considering their position as part of the overall health system they are expressing a minority view. This is reflected in particular in their emphasis on the need to 'create healthcare markets' or to strengthen export prospects in the field of health services defined as an underdeveloped area in terms of exports of services.

In relation to politics and political accountability it is striking that since the mid 1980s the shift towards commercialisation has taken place in a context where centre-right governments have changed the legal framework to enable more commercialisation as part of explicit policy priorities. The centre-left or left-conservative governments have been relatively unengaged, but have legitimated these policies as part of broader sets of processes often in the form of pilot programmes, which have enabled the continuation of the direction of change. This evolution is in part a product of a particular government programme establishing the policy priorities for successive governments, but has to be seen in the context of priorities in health versus priorities in overall policies.

On the other hand, in terms of public participation and the role of users in planning of health services, the policies, discussions and debates remain relatively limited in Finland. Democratic accountability is still dominant in the context of local government elections and the role of municipalities in organising and delivering health services. This remains the case in spite of changes in the municipal legislation and a general emphasis on direct participation and deliberative decision making. Corporate interest groups continue the tradition of being included in consultations and parliamentary hearings as part of the broader policy-making arena. On the practical side, many NGOs find it difficult to comply with government procurement as it treats them in the same terms as private sector corporations and has impacted on their funding; such approaches are at odds with NGOs' traditional emphasis on more co-operative and negotiation-based models (Möttönen and Niemelä 2005).

Conclusion

In Finland public participation and the commercialisation of health services have to a large extent been promoted through different mechanisms and channels. While consumers or customers and their rights might be emphasised in the context of promoting market mechanisms or choice in healthcare, there is less understanding or emphasis on the implications for citizens and their rights. The debates that do occur are framed by constitutional, social and human rights and are championed by different actors than those promoting choice and market mechanisms.

The dominant context for commercialisation in Finland is a historical institutional context in service provision altered through incremental shifts and ideological preferences. The role of government actors, in particular the Ministry of Trade and Industry, Office of Competition and the Ministry of Finance, as active supporters and participants in this process is very apparent. This pressure has been complemented by prominent industry leaning think tanks and a broader emphasis on the productivity and competitiveness of the national economy. Globalisation has had less impact on commercialisation in terms of unavoidable consequences, than it has had on legitimating particular views and providing support for specific ideological preferences. European policies have contributed to the growing commercialisation and changes in the Finnish legal framework. It is in the context of European policies, however, that some of the clearest national policy debates *against* commercialisation and commercially driven health systems have taken place.

The process of reforming public services and healthcare was initially articulated in Finland in the context of local autonomy and democratic accountability, but has since become reframed in the context of a search for productivity, efficiency and an increasing role for other than public sector providers. Furthermore, any consideration of citizen involvement and emphasis has become articulated more in the context of customers and clients, rather than in terms of public participation or deliberative action. In part this is due to the separation of municipal service provision from the accountability for local governance. This new emphasis is also based on the almost sole emphasis on choice and vouchers as mechanisms for realising the patient choice agenda.

The lessons to highlight from Finland are the relevance of decentralisation to the policy dynamics of reforms and, second, the lack of participatory or direct involvement of users in the planning or development of services. Instead choice and consumerist (exit) options of participation dominate and consequently weaken the role of democratic accountability (voice) as services are provided more jointly. The impact of globalisation has become embedded in politics emphasising the technical necessities of globalisation in a context where health services are increasingly considered commercial services or a platform for further 'product' development and innovation. This articulation represents a demarcation of the increasing distance between citizens' views and policy priorities. However, the final lesson is that even if change has become promoted as a technical and administrative measure, politics still matter both at the level of municipalities and in the context of national policies.

9 Healthcare reforms, user involvement and markets in England, Finland and Sweden

Are there common concerns?

In this chapter we draw together the often separate discourses on citizen engagement and patient involvement on one hand and on health systems' reform on the other, and the evidence from the three case studies. Studies on healthcare reforms have tended to focus on particular aspects such as economics, politics or issue of rights from particular perspectives such as law, sociology or political science. We have also been intrigued by the ways in which policy developments and, in particular, commercialisation of healthcare has taken different routes and emphases in the three countries we studied. We are intrigued with the ways that the rhetoric justifying reforms is more amenable to political orientation than the mechanisms adopted to drive the reform agenda and how some policy ideas seem to have diffused faster than others.

We divide this chapter into subsections each of which focuses on a key area that emerged from our critical comparison of the evolution of health policy reforms. We start by discussing the background for policies and the context of health policy making and how these broader undercurrents influenced the policy solutions that emerged in all three countries. We move on to discuss the evolution of patient rights and then continue to explore how decentralisation has interacted with health reform and the trend to primary care led health systems. The next section takes up the issue of policy diffusion and innovation in relation to health reforms before turning to the tensions between patient involvement and choice. We go on to explore how processes of globalisation and Europeanisation shape the health policy space in the three countries before exploring the evolution of health policy apparent in England, Finland and Sweden. However, we begin by elaborating three broad undercurrents that shape the direction of policy change.

The broader undercurrents and policy change

The comparison of policy processes and outcomes across countries always carries a risk of either overstating or understating the influence of international policy transfer. The predominant emphasis in comparative studies has been on the historical and institutional context of changes, which is often more conducive to explaining differences rather than similarities. An emphasis on *leader* and *follower* countries, on the other hand, is not necessarily attuned to national politics and political sensitivities.

One significant undercurrent is the overall emphasis on cost-containment, productivity and efficiency of the public sector as a whole. The initial global wave of healthcare reforms in OECD countries was driven by cost-containment concerns related to what was seen as the inevitable upward spiral of medical costs. These discussions were framed by emerging neo-liberal theories that justified a new public management as typified by Osborne and Gaebler (1992) and the application of Enthoven's managed competition as justification for the purchaser–provider split.

However, in the 1990s an emerging issue in the United Kingdom was the chronic underfunding of the NHS and the necessity of upgrading facilities but to do so in a way that generated increased productivity and shortened waiting lists. On the other hand, in Finland the health system had expanded during the 1980s and therefore the 1990s represented a time of diminishing resources. The political decisions that sought to shrink the public sector were made before the recession in Finland and Sweden, but the health reform processes were significantly affected by a shift in policy priorities as a result of the economic crisis in the early 1990s.

A second undercurrent relates to the establishment of patient rights and the changing role of professionals and professionalism within health systems. This implies an increase in managerial power often exercised through corporate governance mechanisms within healthcare organisations and overseen nationally by protocols and increased regulation. It is also manifested as a growing recognition of more commercial and consumerist priorities within health systems and the development of frameworks under which they could more directly influence health services. This pressure also has implications for citizen and patient interests as they become increasingly interpreted as consumerist rights and a right to choose. On the other hand commercial and provider rights are being increasingly secured through intergovernmental agreements and policies at a European Union and global level. Such shifts frame the debate within the European Union concerning the proposed patient rights in cross-border healthcare directive and the potential cost implications of this for Member States as the accountability for financing remains national and in some health systems local.

The third undercurrent reflects the different and often contested politics between local and national levels of government. In Sweden and Finland cost-containment efforts and processes were implemented through county councils and municipalities, which were responsible for the costs of healthcare. In Finland this also led to a growing share of health funding being gathered through other mechanisms, such as user charges, although user charges were mostly implemented to discourage 'unnecessary' consultations. Furthermore, participation and autonomy at the local level (the localism agenda) were proffered as potential solutions to improve public services by making them more responsive to local communities. However, much of the financial and normative power remained at national level but often outside the health sector. This trend is exacerbated by processes at the European level which the European Commission increasingly seeks to shape health policy.

The need to curb the rising public costs of healthcare

It can be argued that in all three countries health reforms were initially articulated in the context of cost-containment within health systems and core concerns over increasing public sector expenditure and the use of market mechanisms and competition to reduce costs. Inspiration for this form of policy solution came predominantly from United States and in particular the work of Alain Enthoven:

> In an appropriately designed system of fair economic competition among various types of health plan, including traditional insurance and fee-for-service as one option, consumers who join health plans that do a good job of controlling costs would pay lower premiums or receive better benefits. Health plans that do a poor job of controlling costs would lose customers and risk being driven out of business. In the long run, the surviving health plans would be the ones that offer good value to their members. The health system would be transformed, gradually and voluntarily, from today's system with built-in cost-increasing incentives to a system with built-in incentives for customer satisfaction and cost-control.
>
> (Enthoven 1980: 131)

While Enthoven's thinking continued to be reflected in reforms in England, for example, in the work of Julian Le Grand, it is clear that his influence was greatest in the introduction of the so-called internal market reforms initiated during the 1980s and early 1990s. The touchstone of economics and the power of market discipline to drive reform also contributed to Swedish policies in the 1990s and in particular the promotion of planned markets and choice (Blomqvist 2004; Saltman and Otter 1992).

In the United Kingdom the use of competition as a mechanism to lower costs and improve efficiency was initiated during successive Conservative governments under the premiership of Margaret Thatcher and subsequently John Major. In Sweden and Finland this articulation became stronger in the context of the economic crisis in the early 1990s and the recovery measures legitimised the imposition of greater competitiveness within the national economy (Uusitalo 1996; Timonen 2003), and strengthened the position and role of Ministries of Finance in comparison to Ministries of Health and Social Affairs.

In this first phase of reforms, market mechanisms were implemented primarily to improve competitiveness between providers within the health system. The intention was to harness competition to reduce costs or at least limit their growth. In both Finland and Sweden a crucial pressure in defining 'appropriate' healthcare reforms was based on support by government actors outside Ministries of Health rather than within them. As national economic concerns were amplified, the position and reach of the Ministry of the Interior and the Ministries of Finance and Trade and Industry were strengthened. Thus, in Finland it was the Office of Competition which initially called for more competition in healthcare, not the Ministry of Social Affairs and Health.

The emphasis on productivity and efficiency gains as outcomes of competition and the benefits of contracting with private sector providers remains a core principle of health reforms in all three countries. In all three countries arguments promoting markets and competition as the means to generate cost-containment have been based more on expectations than on evidence of outcomes. The organisational changes have remained and, in the case of Finland, strengthened as an outcome of municipal reforms. The consequence has been the creation of an environment for a more contractual structure of healthcare organisations and services.

In all three countries the provision of primary healthcare has become intertwined with the broader public sector reforms and changes in local governance processes. At the same time, changes in hospital governance have been driven more through particular corporatisation processes. In England changes in the structure and organisation of governance and control, including different contractual relationships with GPs have been framed in terms of raising quality and spreading good practice rather than in terms of efficiency and productivity. In Sweden this trend is evident in policies and policy changes relating to family doctors and choice in primary healthcare.

The role of the privately financed commercial health sector or private health insurance companies has been limited in all three countries. In England the use of private companies to provide NHS services has been heavily constrained and mostly limited to specific interventions with large waiting lists. These constraints are beginning to shift as some GP surgeries are beginning to be contracted out. The other space that has been created for private sector actors is as consultants and providers of administrative and strategic support. Increasingly in the English context this is apparent in the new approach to commissioning services (Department of Health 2007; 2008b). While not always made explicit, the implicit assumption has been that increasing productivity to diminish waiting lists might require increased provision. At the same time the private sector was presented as more efficient and a source of inspiration and relevant models for public sector providers. This linked contracting out and competition to a drive for increased service quality and improved performance. The paradox is that in all three countries while cost-containment was the initial argument for change, the lack of success or varying experiences from the use of competition has not resulted in a rolling back of competition, but rather a change in the justification.

The evolution of rights and changing emphasis within health systems

Another key theme that has emerged from our analysis relates to a growing emphasis on patient participation emerging in health policies on the one hand and the establishment of legal rights on the other. The basic starting point in terms of social rights and public participation differs across the countries and relates to broader national policy articulation. In England, with no written constitution, rights of access to healthcare are defined by directives from central government and have been presented in terms of aspirations in the *Patient's Charter* (Department of Health 1991), although current debate over an NHS Constitution (Department of Health 2008c) may alter this situation. Importantly these debates have moved on from defining the obligation of the state, and the NHS organisation, to providing healthcare to suggest a reciprocal relationship of 'rights and obligations'.

In Finland patient rights legislation was pioneering, but is still relatively weak although rights of access to care are also defined in the Finnish Constitution. Rights to access were also further elaborated in relation to the 'care guarantee'. In Sweden the legal basis for patients' rights is weaker than in Finland because of a political preference and tradition of non-legal instruments, for example in the context of the Swedish care guarantee. In the light of the elaboration of non-legal guidance and intervention from central government in England, the Swedish and Finnish health systems seem relatively unregulated.

While the journey towards greater commercialisation and marketisation of health services has taken place in all three countries, national legislation on health-related consumer rights and their relevance to healthcare, including aspects relevant to contractual arrangements in healthcare, seem to have been more of an afterthought. In other words, while the process of commercialisation and contracting out has been envisaged as a solution to the problems of health systems, there has been a lack of focus on the 'dark side' of these arrangements and respective requirements to balance such mechanisms with greater 'consumer' rights. This is an issue in all three countries, where measures to enhance patient rights have not been framed as consumer rights. Such rights are crucially important for patients in the context of providing protection when things go wrong or a provider defaults. This particular area of patient rights is framed instead as the right to complain; the provision of rights of redress, requirements for insurance from providers or implementation of no-faults insurance would be one potential response. While these measures do cover the major problem cases and harm caused to people, they do not address more mundane issues with respect to inadequacy of services or how services are provided. In Finland contracted-out services remained the responsibility of the local government in terms of their content and adequacy. If a private provider who is contracted to provide a public service fails, this does not discharge the responsibility of the municipality for the content and adequacy of the service. Patients who had contracted privately with a default-ing provider would enjoy consumer protection; a protection not extended to patients receiving publicly funded services from the same defaulting provider, but must seek redress through the other avenues.

Primary care: caught between local and national agendas

Another broader undercurrent present in the evolution of health policy is the process of decentralisation and the relationship between local and national policies. In health systems this is further affected by broader debates around strengthening primary healthcare, led initially by the WHO jointly with UNICEF (1978). In England health reforms have at least paid lip-service to this shift in orientation by defining primary care trusts as the purchasers of more than 80 per cent of healthcare services. The ambivalence in central gov-ernment to create opportunities for autonomy and independence has led to conflicting policy measures. Hospitals have been encouraged to become inde-pendent Foundation Trusts and the commissioning of services – the prioriti-sation and purchasing of care for a given population – is now required to include patient and public involvement. Both of these changes have been pre-sented as creating an NHS that is more responsive to local people. Yet, cen-tral government has retained the power to set targets and has established multi-tiered governance arrangements that require far greater information collection and surveillance.

In Sweden and Finland, responsibility for service provision has been decen-tralised, where county councils in Sweden and municipalities in Finland have significant power to decide how services are provided. In Sweden the em-phasis on local services was initially implemented in the context of a trad-itional hospital-based system. This autonomy at county council level led to varied and diverse applications of commercialisation resulting in central government intervention in the context of the so called Stop-Law to halt the threat of selling off public hospitals by some county councils. Decentralisation has increased the complexity of actors and views presented as part of national policies and highlighted the technical impact of political changes. The decentralisation of responsibility for the provision of healthcare has further complicated debates on democratic accountability, local gover-nance and responsiveness to community priorities.

In Finland, for example, the initial establishment of the purchaser–provider split was made in the context of decentralisation policies and not as a health policy. Central government held that while municipalities were responsible for provision of health services, it was also up to them to decide on how they spent their money. The paradox has been that while local gov-ernment autonomy has been emphasised in the governance of health services, other policy measures overseen by other ministries, such as those related to government procurement, have been implemented centrally and enforced on municipalities.

In Sweden and Finland implementation of new public management-related measures in local government have been prominent and extensive and have impacted on an array of public sector services including health. While local government reforms continue to evolve, in England the local government has little formal relationship to, or responsibility for, the organisation or delivery of health services. Thus, the impact of health of such reforms is far clearer in Sweden and Finland where primary healthcare provision and services remain the responsibility of the local government. The importance of decentralisation needs to be set in the context of the redistributive function of health systems and where an emphasis on entrepreneurial aspects of local governance, including the retention of funds may increase inequalities. Decentralisation has implications for equity, which in health systems has to be considered not only between populations but also where they live (Koivusalo *et al.* 2007).

The diffusion and lack of diffusion of ideas and common influences

Internationally, governments and policy makers, share, compare and explore different policy options. This pattern of policy diffusion is particularly evident in the three countries we studied. In many ways England has been a forerunner particularly in terms of the marketisation of health services, and Swedish and Finnish policies have followed. However, the process of health reforms in both Sweden and Finland were initiated very early. In the case of enhancing choice, Sweden was also clearly promoting choice before this was a major policy issue in England or Finland.

Traditionally, Finnish policy reforms have followed Swedish examples, but the reality is more nuanced. It is clear that policy diffusion has taken place, but the policies that emerged have been based on the mediating influence of the national context and political sensibilities. It can also be argued that for some reforms the direction of policy diffusion is not from England to Sweden and on to Finland, but rather from the United States to a number of European countries. The internal market reforms in Sweden and Finland can be seen as a product influenced more by the same ideas that influenced change in England, rather than the experience of implementing internal markets in the NHS.

The importance of the US managed care experience as well as the example of Kaiser Permanente inspired policy interest is visible in all three countries. England was thus not the sole reference point for Sweden and Finland. The focus and promotion of consumer-driven or consumer-led models and vouchers provides another clear example of US influence on health policy reforms. Models of health savings accounts have also been taken up in both Sweden and Finland by think tanks and representatives of business and industry (TIMBRO 2005; Korkman *et al.* 2007).

On the other hand, not all policy issues gain ground in other contexts. The Private Finance Initiative, a form of public–private partnership that combines capital investment and service operation (Pollock 2004; Her Majesty's

Treasury 2003), for example, remained almost exclusively an issue specific to the United Kingdom and within the UK mostly limited to England. While some enthusiasts, at least in Finland, explored this approach, it has not – at least not so far – become financially attractive in either Sweden or Finland. The absence of traction for the Private Finance Initiative approach in Swedish and Finnish health policy making has meant that we have only touched on it in very limited ways in this book.

The Patient's Charter is another example of a policy that emerged in the UK but was exported. The initial aim and implementation of the policy, however, may alter when it is transplanted to a different context. The Patient Charter that emerged in Finland was moulded by the Finnish and Swedish orientation towards contractual agreements in service provision and emerged with a far more technical emphasis (Haverinen 1999) than the aspirational orientation that typified the Citizen's Charter initiative in the UK (Tritter 1994).

The diffusion of policies and policy ideas also follows vectors established by particular key actors or organisations. The role of Alain Enthoven and Kaiser Permanente has already been identified, but the increasing part played by international management consultant firms has created another transmission route for certain types of policy concepts (Saint-Martin 1998). The implications of this increased role, has been likened by some to a transfer of power and the emergence of a new form of governance, 'consultocracy'. As Hodge and Bowman explain, 'the "Consultocracy" alludes to the increasing influence of private sector management consultants on the reform and agenda processes of the public sector' (2006: 99). Judgement of the role that consultants play has varied from viewing them as constructive advisors to the emergence of a non-elected elite (Lapsley and Oldfield 2001). There is no doubt that management consultants have had a significant impact in shaping policy in all three countries, but arguably this has been greatest in England. As Bloomfield and Danieli reflect,

> changes in the NHS are largely a result of government policies, but management consultants represent important purveyors of these ideas . . . as intermediaries, they are not neutral conduits but important actors, whose role is constitutive of some of the changes taking place.
>
> (Bloomfield and Danieli 1995: 34)

What is far more obscure is the process of selecting management consultants and what, if any, conflicts of interest are embedded in their advice.

Professional associations, unions, and particularly medical unions, are important actors in shaping health policy and may serve as both conduits and sources for policy ideas. Private sector doctors have been an important part of the medical association lobby both in Finland and Sweden, whereas in England the stance of the British Medical Association has been more mixed; both *Keep our NHS Public* (2009) and *Doctors for Reform* (Reform 2008) have followings within the British Medical Association, but support opposite positions and proffer alternative solutions to the problems of the NHS.

User involvement and patient choice

The implementation of user involvement as a deliberative process and part of services planning and improvement is an area which has been taken much further in England than in either Sweden or Finland. What is striking is the lack of focus on direct participatory mechanisms within health policies in Sweden and Finland. While Sweden in particular has a tradition of inclusive and open policy making through committee work and consultations, there seems to be far less focus on user involvement as part of the development and planning of services. This is apparent in many ways, but particularly clearly with respect to how users of health services and user-led organisations participate – or do not participate – in policy development, service prioritisation, organisation or improvement. In Sweden and Finland the focus on empowering patients seems to be, on the one hand, on the enhancement of individual patient choice and, on the other, on ensuring forms of democratic decision making through municipalities or county councils. In Sweden a different phenomena has emerged with the emergence of health interest political parties, which seem to reinforce a kind of populist agenda on healthcare.

The utility of public participation in deliberative processes to shape policy was familiar to our respondents in Sweden and Finland. Explaining the English situation of formal legally sanctioned patient and public involvement mechanisms that require engagement of service users as part of service improvement and development was far more difficult for them to comprehend or identify comparable examples in Sweden or Finland. Our focus was not merely on the existence of 'lay' members on hospital boards or the influence of patient groups in consultations, but rather a broader understanding of the importance of user involvement and engagement for health services planning and development. Our conclusions are that such a role for patients and the public is not systematically present either in Finland or in Sweden and indeed it is unclear whether there is any pressure to create the space for this to occur.

Swedish policies have more explicitly and over a longer period embraced commercialisation and patient choice than in either England or Finland, although not necessarily more effectively. The expansion of patient choice in the Swedish health system has been slow and as a steering mechanism has been considered a policy failure (Winblad 2007). The current government, however, has significantly advanced the choice agenda with the clear aim of enhancing individual patient choice across the country. The efforts in Finland are also geared towards legislative changes to provide scope for patient choice within the health system as well as increase the use of service vouchers in municipalities. The focus on 'free choice' and vouchers in Sweden and Finland seems to emphasise a far more individualised 'choice' than in England. In England patient choice has been advanced, but is limited to the choice of the location of service delivery. In effect, choice is primarily a mechanism not to empower individual patients, but to drive competition between

NHS hospitals. It is unclear whether there is political will to drive the choice agenda further, and the strengthening of the requirement for commissioners to consult with local people – to encourage responsive local communities as part of a broader localisation agenda – may limit further the elaboration of patient choice.

Globalisation and Europeanisation

The role of European Union policies and their relevance to national health systems is recognised in all three countries, but considered least relevant in England. In Sweden the assumption is that national policy priorities should prevail, whereas in Finland national policies seem to make an early adjustment to European requirements on the basis of views on the formal legal implications of the European policies. It is worth noting that our study focused on England but that in terms of the European Union the United Kingdom is the Member State.

After the initial series of European Court of Justice judgments relating to healthcare there was a common concern across a number of Member States of the potential consequences of expansion of internal markets and the ways in which they would influence health systems. This has also been reflected in the European Council statement on Common Values and Principles in EU Health Systems (Council of the European Union 2006).

Finland, Sweden and the United Kingdom were also active in relation to the proposed new Constitutional Treaty of the European Union with the aim of limiting the influence of internal market rules on national health systems. However, it is unclear to what extent cooperation and exchange across countries has taken place after changes in government in Finland and Sweden. Decentralisation in the United Kingdom is likely to affect positions in Brussels, where English, Scottish and Welsh health interests are dealt alongside national industry interests. Similarly in Finland and Sweden, the separation of responsibility for the delivery of health services to municipalities in Finland and county councils in Sweden distances them from European Union decision making, although there are channels for cooperation and representation for local governments within the European Union. However, decisions about the free movement of patients within the European Union, for instance, are based on the position and negotiations by national, central government. This creates a particular form of governance gap that reinforces the existing tension between those who have the responsibility for organising and delivering health services and those who set the context within which delivery occurs. The challenge in Finland and particularly in Sweden, in relation to the European policies and perhaps globalisation, is the extent to which existing light regulatory approaches based on information steering and other 'soft' measures are vulnerable to the harder legalistic regulatory measures that are part of commercial service sector processes.

The role and relevance of globalisation and European policies to national health systems in England, Sweden and Finland seems rather paradoxical. While the health systems in all three countries provide good value for money in terms of their performance, the politics of globalisation exert pressure towards greater individualised and commercialised health service provision. European policies do not require patient choice as a primary driver within a health system, but merely arrangement to accommodate mobility of patients residing in other European Union countries. Yet, when patient choice becomes a mechanism to drive commercial access to health systems then governments could rightly claim that it potentially endangers the financial sustainability of their health systems. Historically, the health systems within the three countries have been successful in containing costs, thus the reason for the current moves towards plurality and choice in service provision is more likely to be based on ideological, commercial and industrial interests. This is particularly clear in Finland, where surveys indicate public support for the welfare state and critical views towards commercialisation of health services (Forma *et al.* 2007b).

The division between the United Kingdom and European interests is also apparent in the establishment of a new NHS European Office in Brussels in 2007. The role of European policies and in particular European social policies has different impacts on individual Member States. In the United Kingdom the debates concerning European Union policies are embedded in the avoidance of social and employment directives, and in particular the Working Time Directive, which in part reflects a hangover from the Thatcher era. On the other hand, in Sweden, and especially in Finland, the approach to this directive is much more accommodating. While the Working Time Directive was raised in our interviews in England, it was not brought up as strongly in Finland or Sweden.

In Finland and Sweden the emphasis on legal requirements for government procurement shapes the context and scope in which healthcare reforms, and contracting out, takes place. Compliance with the EU Directive on Government procurement is not required for health services, yet Finland chose to interpret and apply the legal framework more broadly. In England the emphasis on contracts and commercialisation has emerged from national policy choices. It is likely that the early adoption of more European Union compatible requirements for government procurement across public sectors in Finland and Sweden have raised concerns that may emerge in the NHS in the future. In England, the implications of competitive compulsory tendering have not been of equal concern, although there have been calls for greater transparency in awarding contracts to the private sector that have been seen as too lucrative.

Bringing the politics back in: the evolution of health policy in Sweden, Finland and England

Shifts in the political stance of the party in power account for the development and elaboration of some health policies and can be explained in part by traditional party policies and changes in right-centre-left governments. But whatever the political orientation of the government, similar mechanisms – encouraging competition between providers, promoting patient choice – are apparent in all three countries but often legitimated with very different rhetoric. The definition of policy 'solutions' and policy 'innovations' is perhaps explained by shifts in power from Health Ministries to Ministries of Finance and Trade and Industry. This reconfiguration of the power hierarchy in central government creates the opportunity to extend influence over health policy options and is particularly apparent in Finland and Sweden and gained ground as a result of the economic crises in the early 1990s.

In England the reforms in the late 1990s were linked to significant increases in funding and it was in this context that patient choice and involvement became possible; without surplus in the system all that can be accomplished is choosing between waiting lists. But the consequence of the scale of additional funding was a greater say by the Treasury in how accountability for spending – performance measures – was implemented.

The evolution towards more market orientation in health services in all three countries seems to have been continuous since the late 1980s. However, this process is sensitive to political shifts, and pro-market policies have greater emphases, and was more actively implemented under centre-right governments in Finland and Sweden; governments that also seem to put less emphasis on collective risk sharing and the public health aspects of health systems. In contrast, the politics of New Labour in England were not directly opposed to market solutions and were concerned with health inequalities, but could not find a 'third way' that would generate the centralised governance and accountability demanded by the Treasury in the context of significant public investment.

While the welfare states in Sweden and Finland in many ways have been more extensive, the NHS with the support of health professionals dedicated to a common set of values seems to have maintained, at least until recently, greater resilience towards commercialisation. In Finland and Sweden, medical doctors as a group have been more supportive of commercialisation and have sought to engage with this agenda through corporate practices and corporatisation, yet do not necessarily grasp the potential consequences on professional autonomy and the shift of power to managers and corporate executives, a pattern that has become so apparent in the examples of Health Maintenance Organisations in the United States.

Conclusion

Instead of seeing England as the leader of health policy reforms and Finland and Sweden as followers, it would be more appropriate to view each of these countries as having faced similar political and policy pressures. The policy responses to these pressures as well as continued European Union integration are a series of health system modifications that, however, must be understood in their national institutional and historical context. In this respect some aspects of policy measures were implemented earlier, as part of decentralisation in Sweden and Finland and others are now being implemented for a second time, such as the purchaser–provider split in Finland.

Policy transfer and diffusion is not the sole preserve of the health sector, but takes place across other disciplines and through other sectors. Furthermore, as a large proportion of the healthcare industry is global, their efforts to influence policies at a national level are based on global policy interests. It is in this context that the evolution of health policy and health systems in England, Finland and Sweden need to be understood. In an arena where commercialisation is driven by global and European interests it is unlikely that patient and public involvement in health systems can remain local. However, globalisation as such does not imply that national health systems could not resist external pressures towards commercialisation, despite the overlap they may have with some domestic interests.

The message of this comparative analysis is that the current process of commercialisation and patient choice in the three countries should be set in the context of politics and values rather than a value-free technical framework. Patient choice is not synonymous with patient empowerment let alone patient and public involvement. Patient choice is also not ideologically neutral, but tends to be promoted within a particular set of policy priorities that promote individualisation of financial burden and the dismantling of collective risk and resource sharing within health systems. While in all three systems contractualisation and commercialisation has taken place, it has not been uniform and is unlikely to be so in the future. The starting points for health policy reform have not been similar, nor the menu from which policy choices were selected; this makes it easy to dismiss the commonalities that remain.

In all three countries there is a risk that patient choice becomes the main mechanism for participation and 'empowerment'. Yet patient and public involvement can be seen as a partial antidote to the value-free individualism that appears to be reinforced by the patient choice and commercialisation policy agendas. It seeks instead to generate, at a local level, within communities a relationship between those who provide healthcare services and those who benefit directly and indirectly. It is an approach that is premised not on consumerism and the purchasing by patients of healthcare services but rather the generation of accountability for the way services are prioritised, organised and delivered. It offers the expertise that comes from being the object of care and validates the way individual professionals deliver their care. Patient and public involvement has the potential to create greater co-production of health and wellbeing and build the social capital that is needed to call local providers to account for meeting local health needs and addressing local inequalities. The pressures for and aims of commercialisation are often in conflict with health policy priorities. Governments thus need to consider the purpose of health systems and develop policies that reinforce rather than undermine those aims.

10 Any road will do if you don't know where to go

Conclusions and future prospects

It is hard to argue against more effective and efficient use of public resources to deliver healthcare. It is difficult to be against mechanisms to promote quality improvement and innovation through competition between healthcare providers within a publicly funded health system and the drawing of insights from diverse private sector providers. The promotion of greater transparency and availability of information to enable patients to make better choices about their own healthcare seems a worthy intention.

Yet, none of these aims engage with issues of social solidarity and public accountability. The definition of the problems within healthcare and the solutions that are proferred are all within a particular framework – healthcare markets. The framing of healthcare reforms in terms that give primacy to individual consumers fails to reflect the reality of how healthcare is delivered or how patients make decisions about their own care. Healthcare is increasingly the product of multi-disciplinary teams whether working in a hospital cancer clinic or a primary care health centre. Economically inspired rational choice models may provide an excellent basis for *post hoc* explanation but they are far less effective as models of individual action (Archer and Tritter 2000). When faced with a diagnosis patients reflect on their treatment options not in isolation but through engagement with their social network; the views of their partner, family, parents and friends all shape healthcare decisions.

In this concluding chapter we reflect on our analysis of the impact of globalisation and markets on redefining patients as individual consumers and raise a series of implications for the evolutionary process we have documented. We suggest critical issues in relation to the future of health systems in these countries that have broader implications for other countries and other health systems. Health policy reforms over almost two decades have embraced markets-based competition and promoted consumerism and diversity of providers. The future of health systems in terms of sustainability and the future for patients in terms of equity are in part a product of the continued disputation between the rights of citizens, the role of the state and the desire for profit. We also return to a discussion of globalisation and the need for an improved articulation of the common challenges to health systems.

In this book we have sought to track policy developments and changes in England, Finland and Sweden in comparison to each other, but also within the context of the European Union and as subject to the guidance and influence of international actors such as the WHO, WTO and OECD. We have focused on health policy and the shaping of health policy space rather than implementation. Policy ideas in health do not emerge merely from exchange and learning between health policy makers but are a product of a far more diverse arena inhabited by policy makers, professionals, for-profit and non-profit organisations, professional advisers and pundits as well as the convoluted political process.

In this context it is interesting to go back to the early visionaries promoting planned markets in Sweden. In a study published in 1992 two scholars of healthcare reforms, particularly in Sweden, Richard Saltman and Casten van Otter, not only established the notion of public competition in ways which could be accommodated by social democratic governments, but also further emphasised the importance of democracy and centrality of patient choice in a new role as a means of *expanding democracy*. The focus on planned market reforms in their book covering the United Kingdom, Finland and Sweden argues that 'public competition's emphasis on empowering patients enhances the democratic character of both healthcare system and society overall' (Saltman and Otter 1992: 153).

They also predict that a new policy paradigm will emerge that will generate major structural change throughout publicly operated health systems, a consequence that in hindsight appears to be all but inevitable. As more than 15 years have passed since the publication of their book, it is clear we need to agree that a new paradigm has emerged; however, we are less sure about the extent to which this has served the ends and means that were initially intended. Despite their discarding of the 'atomised notion of empowerment' (Saltman and Otter 1992: 153) that relied on fixed price vouchers, it is exactly these policy responses, vouchers, that are emerging as the next policy option in the name of enhancing patient rights.

The myth of neutrality

In the three countries the articulation of health systems and planned market has been based on, first, the maintenance of public financing and second, the irrelevance of whether public or private sector organisation provides services. In the light of globalisation and the emerging regulatory frameworks, governing the market for services through international organisations, agreements and treaties as well as emerging emphases on government procurement rules appear to matter. Therefore how services are organised and regulated globally, at a European level and nationally, matters now and will matter more in the future.

As services are being out-sourced, health systems enter more deeply into a new regulatory context, which is framed by internal markets, competition and procurement laws within the European Union. This has implications in relation for fragmentation and continuity of care. In this broader framework the task of regulation on the basis of health policy priorities, principles and values, such as equity, solidarity and universality, becomes more challenging. However, this also applies to the scope of national policy space to ensure financial sustainability within health systems as well as the kind of mechanisms used to limit costs.

In the light of our findings we are concerned with the narrowing of participation and democratic accountability simply to an emphasis on choice and vouchers as the primary means of empowering patients. The proponents of patient empowerment now come from the corporate think tanks and employers' associations with visions of a 'win-win situation' where low public costs are combined with patient choice and more individualised financing of health systems accommodating better mobility within nations and across Europe. It is in this context that the emphasis on 'money following patients' is problematic.

It is clear that in all three health systems a particular discourse is opening in relation to increasing user cost sharing on the basis of top-ups and additional costs that patients should be able to choose to pay if they want private sector services or costlier medicines. The choice to pay more is not a neutral choice and is likely to lead towards greater cost sharing by users until complementary insurances or other mechanisms are found and will almost certainly have regressive consequences in terms of inequality.

This situation, we claim, is emerging due to three kinds of economic interests. First, the idea of health services as a commercial sector with prospects of creating new business opportunities and economic development within nation states. Second, powerful buyers, like the NHS, compromise the scope for industry to set prices for new technologies and medicines. Third, there is a need to keep public expenditure low and to seek health system models that do not increase the use of public resources. The result is a conceptualisation of service users as individually empowered patients managing their healthcare utilisation through patient choice and financing mechanisms, such as health savings accounts or additional private health insurance. Health or medical savings accounts could also benefit the financial markets more broadly in the same way as pension reforms have led to a boon for the financial service sector.

The problem is, of course, that while these models might appeal to those who believe in market mechanisms in healthcare, these models tend to undermine the collective risk and resource sharing and cross-subsidisation that is the premise in most publicly funded health systems. Such an approach would also provide clear incentives for providers and insurers to more actively choose patients. The outcome is a health system where public sector costs are lower and more predictable while private costs would be higher. The solutions proposed are not very 'citizen friendly' as they discard a central source of social solidarity and introduce mechanisms that are certain to drive increased inequality and cost sharing by users. Longer-term concerns also apply as the resulting polarisation of a national health service leads to a system for those who can pay and an impoverished service for those who cannot. The latter becomes a public health service that disproportionally has the responsibility for treating those who are more ill, more deprived and older.

The emergence of new proponents for patient rights

As many of the new proponents of choice seem to come more from the side of employers, providers, free-market and industry oriented think tanks, these tend to represent particular interests and values within the society. While in England medical doctors have been more sceptical, in Finland and Sweden medical doctors have embraced the choice agenda as it also opens the scope to choose patients. As choice is promoted as a blanket resolution to inefficiencies and quality concerns of public services, this tends to be based on assumptions of inherent capacities of private sector to improve services provision. Yet looking at the health system as a whole there is no evidence to indicate this. Furthermore, equity in access to care both across individuals and geograph-ical regions implies that choice would require balancing measures. While choice is typically discussed in terms of actions by patients, it is clear that the legitimation of choice opens up the scope for providers to choose their patients.

It is striking in the context of the three countries we studied that there is no apparent pressure from citizens for increased choice. In Finland, the surveys point to more critical attitudes by members of the public towards commercialisation and support to publicly financed health services. In Sweden, where choice has reportedly been welcomed by citizens, increased choice is not necessarily at the top of the list on what people want from health services. In fact in the recent WHO survey on responsiveness 3 per cent of Swedes and 6 per cent of Finns considered choice as the most important aspect of non-clinical care. In the survey, prompt attention, dignity and communication were clearly more important for the respondents (Valentine *et al.* 2008). The crucial question is to what extent current policies also overstate the importance of choice in comparison to other aspects of healthcare.

We need to ask where the push for patient choice comes from. While it is reasonable to expect that some choice should be accommodated within health systems, the emphasis on patient choice as a steering mechanism, or fundamental principle, to be extended throughout Europe is more problematic. The emphasis on patient choice also tends to undermine population-based approaches to public health and health policy. While some emphasis is emerging on more individualised mechanisms to tackle public health issues through individual savings accounts or higher premiums for unhealthy lifestyles, there are better and less ethically contentious ways to tackle these challenges.

The dark side of choice

It is also necessary to consider the 'dark side' of patient choice that extends beyond the ordinary concerns over equity and cost escalation. If patient choice is considered an inherently good thing, and important for the values that underpin the operation of health systems, then we need to be serious about clarifying the scope of patient choice that is provided. The capacity to exert choice as a rational consumer is based on information. To make patient choice operate effectively we need to be clear about the limits and scope of the information to enable an informed choice. More importantly we need to recognise and resist the ways that industry interests use information provision as a means of creating demand – and attracting and selecting more 'profitable' patients. Furthermore, we are likely to face constraints in terms of the kind of information that should be provided to the public domain of corporate operations and what can be considered as confidential due to its commercial value.

One purpose of health systems financing and organisation has been to liberate patients from *choices which they should not need to make*. These dilemmas occur when the costs of intervention are extremely heavy and overwhelm the capacity of any but the most wealthy patients to pay; should patients in this situation sell assets or mortgage their house to access a treatment advertised as a cure? Such dilemmas are further complicated by the evidence base used to justify claims of efficacy. How much are people willing to pay for hope? The nature of health savings account would present additional dilemmas as they provide incentives to refuse treatment where saved funds can be transferred or inherited; for example, a grandmother with an account that is still in surplus falls ill and might decline care so that the resources can be used by her grandson.

In both Sweden and Finland there is a lack of recognition of the potential equity and cost implications of the expansion of choice. Those who promote choice and competition tend to automatically assume that market forces will resolve such issues. In England cost sharing by users still remains more modest as choice has been more strictly governed and regulated, but becomes a real concern in the context of the emphasis of European policies on patient mobility.

The real issue is that, whether we like it or not, the promotion of patient choice is and will always be limited by resources as well as professional and knowledge-based assessments of what kind of care should and can be provided within a public system. Choice is never free and the development of voucher schemes and the direction of European policies suggest that choice will also in future come with a hefty price – financial, social and ethical.

Social, patient and consumer rights in healthcare

The difference between social and individual rights has been central to health policy debates. What has emerged is an understanding that while social rights are enjoyed collectively and cover aspects such as access to care and provision of adequate health services, individual rights to patient care are more readily expressed in absolute terms and can be made enforceable on behalf of individual patients.

There is a clear confusion in terms of what these different rights imply in practice. Health systems are needs-based, not structured around 'wants'. Social rights are set in a broader context in which health systems operate as well as the basis of their function. Proponents of patient choice use the language of rights. However, as far as we know, international declarations and charters on human and social rights do not include patient choice as a right. On the other hand, the initial context in which rights to health were established suggests three other points of interest:

> The extension to all peoples of the benefits of medical, psychological and related knowledge is essential to the fullest attainment of health. Informed opinion and active co-operation on the part of the public are of the utmost importance in the improvement of the health of the people. Governments have the responsibility for the health of their peoples which can be fulfilled only by the provision of adequate health and social measures.
>
> (WHO 1948: 2)

In Finland the real challenge to the rights to access care is related to challenges of provision in remote geographical areas and the underlying inequalities, neither of which will be ameliorated by enhancing patient choice. In Sweden, new health reforms and the promotion of patient choice are generating more critical insights. Dahlgren (2008) has pointed out that as part of the Health and Medical Services Act 1982, the overall objectives of the health system are still to provide equal care for equal need across the entire population regardless of age, sex, ethnic background, socioeconomic position or economic resources. For Sweden it can be argued that the *principles* that underpin the health system are likely to be in conflict with the policies promoting patient *rights to choose*.

This point is also important with respect to the European Council Statement on common values and principles (Council of the European Union 2006). The values and principles, such as universality and solidarity, enshrined in the Statement are in conflict with the right to free choice of service provider within Europe approach that the Commission is proposing (European Commission 2008a), as well as application of internal markets rules as the basis of this proposal. The explanatory part of the European Council statement elaborates what these values imply:

> The overarching values of universality, access to good quality care, equity and solidarity, have been widely accepted in the work of different EU institutions. Together they constitute a set of values that are shared

across Europe. Universality means that no-one is barred access to healthcare; solidarity is closely linked to the financial arrangement of our national health systems and the need to ensure accessibility to all; equity relates to equal access according to need, regardless of ethnicity, gender, age, social status or ability to pay.

(Council of the European Union 2006: 2)

Changing realities in health systems

There are resonant and creative links between the knowledge and experience, and the theoretical and normative concerns of the healthcare systems examined in this book. These include preoccupations with managing complex systems with multiple goals through cross-cutting and multi-level scalar governance, organisational innovation, the drive for citizen-centred governance embedded within pluralist approaches to expertise, unpacking the intended and unintended consequences of modernisation, and leveraging sustainability at the local level – all set within economic constraints.

But there are also core structural and cultural differences that distinguish these systems as particular, situated and individual. For example, England is far advanced in policy articulation and operationalisation of public and patient involvement, whereas in Finland there is less if any focus on this issue, in spite of efforts to address issues of patient rights and complaints. The political and emotional commitment to the NHS as a defining cultural institute is apparent across England and the UK. In Sweden and Finland the welfare state garners similar broad popular support, however, in both countries there is less clearly a sense of the health system as a social institution. In Finland private practice has also remained beside the public sector. However, what is changing is the increasing *commercialisation* of both the private and public sectors as service providers; small private group practices have merged or joined to form larger chains with multinational ownership.

It is also important to consider the impact of managerialism on health professionals as part of health reform processes. In Finland the growth of management has been slower, resulting in the retention of health professional leadership in health services. The growth of managerialism and use of management consultants, however, is apparent in shaping the Finnish and Swedish healthcare reforms. The use of external consults is far less prominent than in England or the NHS, where attention to the wide use of consultants and their power has generated criticism (see e.g. Pollock 2004; Craig 2006).

However, while the growing role for managers and consultants has been a means to tackle professional dominance within the health sector, the results may also have contributed to a process of the decline of health expertise amongst those developing and implementing health policies. The often stated problem in contracting out and using competition in health services is the lack of know-how, yet the longer-term problem within the public sector is not the lack of legal, managerial and business expertise for successful contracting out, but whether such an emphasis also pushes out public health and health service expertise. The expanding role for management consultants can, and should, be seen as part of globalisation processes and in particular the globalisation of ideas and practices. The accommodation of this channel for ideas and influence is grounded in the application of new public management practices.

Globalisation, Europeanisation and commercialisation

Globalisation contributes to pressure on public financing and the scope of taxation. However, these pressures do not necessarily require, or may even contrast with, the promotion of the commercialisation of healthcare. Globalisation may empower those who seek markets in healthcare as well as provides a means for enhancing liberalisation, but *it cannot be seen as requiring the commercialisation of health systems*. Instead, globalisation is often a conveni-ent excuse for commercialisation but decisions to pursue this agenda are political.

The creation of healthcare markets is a process where the commodification of health needs to be supported, articulated and marketed. In this context the drive towards transparency, measurement and the harmonisation of quality indicators is important for market creation and corporate involvement in the provision of healthcare. One aspect of this is the application of diagnostic related groups (DRG) to create a 'currency' enabling trade in health services. Blomgren and Sundén (2008) quote the CEO of Capio, a private healthcare company, envisioning the DRGs as the Euro of healthcare. While harmonisation of quality standards, measurement and transparency seem neutral aims for European policies, these form a part of a broader political context and policy making that promotes the commodification of healthcare and the basis for a 'level' market place.

The emphasis on public financing and primary focus on provision is reflected as part of the public contract markets. However, the exploration of new ways to provide services and the scope for commercialisation takes place in a broader political context. Governments need to be aware of the consequences of this for the return to public provision in the context of global regulatory measures that are securing the rights of providers. While Finland and Sweden have kept health services outside the General Agreement on Trade in Services (GATS), it is clear that many aspects relating to the free movement of services within the internal markets in the European Union will raise similar issues and concerns. European Union Member States can no longer ignore this process, but measures proposed by the European Commission, whether by DG Sanco or DG Employment, seem to enhance rather than limit these developments or mitigate their impact.

The role of internal markets, European Union treaties and trade agreements is, however, often interpreted more tightly than is necessary. This is apparent in the way that Finland adjusted government procurement law.

European Union treaties are negotiated treaties and not 'natural laws'; areas and measures can be included or excluded from internal markets if necessary. However, such actions require active, consistent and European-wide, or in the case of trade agreements, bilateral or global, cooperation. In comparison to globalised industries, national health administrations have far less engagement with treaties and often have little scope to make the case for national health policy space. The case we have raised in respect to the draft Constitutional Treaty illustrates the limited scope for such actions, even though this did not result in appropriate amendments. The emphasis of common values by the European Council can be seen as part of the same process of common concerns. These common concerns are in part driven by an understanding of health and how health systems work. However, the ways in which these values and principles are interpreted is also shaped by political priorities.

Politics matter

Sweden in particular has been long presented as a social-democratic state with broad support for an extensive welfare state. This is still reflected in the ways in which public financing is, and has been, the starting point for any reforms. However, party politics also matter. In Finland the Ministry of Social Affairs and Health did less to actively promote market-oriented reforms under the social-democratic government, but with a change of government new policies emerged and also a more active role for the Ministry. In many ways both Sweden and Finland are currently embracing patient choice and the liberalisation of health services through vouchers far more prominently than England.

The arguments in favour of commercialisation have, in particular, in Finland been technical and framed by a lack of alternatives to support the welfare state. Yet on the basis of what is known about commercialisation of healthcare, the current policies appear to reflect an ideological preference in government rather than popular demand. Furthermore, there is a danger that with an emerging interest in the commercial and export opportunities in health services, health systems become assessed and prioritised primarily as another commercial sector within the society.

Conclusion

In this book we have focused on citizen's rights, public participation and markets in healthcare. Our analysis indicates that in spite of the different origins of the legal 'rights' based discourse and the market models legitimated through economics that have driven healthcare reforms over the last two decades, these two have become mixed in articulating patient choice emerging as a driving force for contemporary health reforms. However, this emphasis undermines the broader context in which social and human rights are defined as well as principles and values underpinning the health systems in England, Finland and Sweden. The danger is that patient choice will be reframed as a right undermining broader-based social rights and displacing principles of solidarity and equity in access to health services.

The promotion of patient choice has taken place in all three countries in a context of the commercialisation of service provision within a publicly funded health system. It is necessary to consider where and what kind of ideas shape the ways in which services are provided and in particular the broader implications of the drive towards more individualised forms of service provision and financing.

Patient and public involvement emphasises dialogue between communities and those who plan and provide services on their behalf. This dialogue is premised on the expertise that the experience of healthcare brings to improving the quality and organisation of health services. Further it creates an accountability mechanism by expecting the justification for what and how services are provided in relation to the needs of the local community and their expression of those needs. There is a danger that patient choice is presented as a form of involvement and the aggregation of individual patient choices becomes a proxy for the involvement of patients and the public in a community.

Finally, we want to emphasise the scope and nature of national policy space that is and needs to be available for health. Globalisation does not require the commercialisation of health systems, even though it does enhance and enable commercialisation. Benefits to the economy and to commercial actors are different aims than improving the health and wellbeing of a population and providing care on the basis of need regardless of the ability to pay. European Union treaties and global agreements on trade are not natural laws or the results of evolutionary forces, but based on negotiation, political priorities and vested interests. Values, principles and politics matter and should emphasise voice more than choice.

Bibliography

Active Citizenship Network (2002) *European Charter of Patient Rights*, Rome: Active Citizenship Network.

Adlung, R. (2006) 'Public services and the GATS', *Journal of International Economic Law*, 9(2): 455–485.

Aho, J. (2004) *Puun ja kuoren välissä*, Valtakunnallinen potilasasiamiesselvitys. Lapin lääninhallituksen julkaisusarja 2004: 8, Rovaniemi: Lapin Lääninhallitus.

Allen, C. (2003) 'Desperately seeking fusion: on "joined-up thinking", "holistic practice" and the *new* economy of welfare professional power', *British Journal of Sociology*, 54 (2): 287–306.

Altenstetter, C. and Busse, R. (2005) 'Healthcare reform in Germany: patchwork change within established governance structures', *Journal of Health Politics, Policy and Law*, 30 (1–2): 121–142.

American Medical Association (AMA) (2008) 'New AMA guidelines on medical tourism', http://www.ama-assn.org/ama1/pub/upload/mm/31/medicaltourism.pdf (accessed 23 July 2008).

Andersen, R., Smedby, B. and Vågerö, D. (2001) 'Cost-containment, solidarity and cautious experimentation: Swedish dilemmas', *Social Science and Medicine*, 52: 1195–1204.

Anell, A. (1996) 'The monopolistic integrated model and healthcare reform: the Swedish experience', *Health Policy*, 37(1): 19–33.

Ansvarskomitte (2007) *Hallbar samhalls organisation med utvecklingskraft*, SOV 200: 10, Stockholm: Government of Sweden.

Appelstrand, M. (2002) 'Participation and societal values: the challenge for lawmakers and policy practitioners', *Forest Policy and Economics*, 4 (4): 281–290.

Appleby, J., Harrison, A. and Devlin, N. (2003) *What is the Real Cost of More Patient Choice?*, London: Kings Fund.

Archer, M. and Tritter, J. (eds) (2000) *Rational Choice Theory: Resisting Colonisation*, London: Routledge.

Armingeon, K. and Beyeler, M. (eds) (2004) *The OECD and European Welfare States*, Cheltenham: Edward Elgar.

Arnstein, S. (1969) 'A ladder of citizen participation', *Journal of the American Institute of Planners*, 35(4): 216–224.

Ashton, J. and Seymour, D. (1988) *The New Public Health*, Milton Keynes: Open University Press.

Avon, Somerset and Wiltshire Cancer Services (2006) 'Annual Report' http://www.aswcs.nhs.uk/AnnualReport.pdf (accessed 5 July 2008).

Bäckström, U., Sörman, H. and Ekström, G. (2008) 'Letter to Europarliament' http://kikaren.skl.se/artikel.asp?C=406&A=56009 (accessed 12 December 2008).

Baggott, R. (2000) 'Understanding the New Public Health: towards a policy analysis', in A. Hann (ed.) *Analysing Health Policy*, Aldershot: Ashgate Publishing.

—— (2004) *Health and Health Care in Britain*, Basingstoke: Palgrave Macmillan.

Balducci, A. and Fareri, P. (1998) 'Consensus-building, urban planning policies, and the problem of scale: examples from Italy', in L. J. O'Toole Jr., D. Huitema and F. H. J. M. Coenen (eds) *Participation and the Quality of Environmental Decision-Making*, Dordrecht: Kluwer Academic Publishers.

Bang, H. (2004) 'Culture governance, governing self reflexive modernity', *Public Administration*, 82(1): 157–190.

Barley, V., Daykin, N., Evans, S., McNeill, J., Palmer, N., Rimmer, J., Sanidas, M., Turton, P. and Tritter, J. (2003) *Developing and Evaluating Best Practice for User Involvement in Cancer Services: Final Report* (Department of Health Grant No. 370051), Bristol: Avon, Somerset and Wiltshire Cancer Services.

Barnard, C. (2007) *The Substantive Law of the EU: The Four Freedoms*, Oxford: Oxford University Press.

Barnes, M. and Prior, D. (1995) 'Spoilt for choice? How consumerism can disempower public service users', *Public Money and Management*, 13(3): 53–58.

Barron, J. (2008) Debate in the House of Commons, *Hansard*, 10 June, column 50WH.

Bell, S., Brada, M., Coombes, C., Miles, B., Morris, E., Richards, M. and Tritter, J. (1996) *"Patient-Centred Cancer Services?" What Patients Say*, Oxford: National Cancer Alliance.

Beresford, P. (2007) 'A matter of choice', *Society Guardian* 30 May, http://www.guardian.co.uk/society/2007/may/30/publicservices.politics (accessed 15 April 2009).

Bergmark, Å. (2008) 'Market reforms in Swedish healthcare: normative reorientation and welfare state sustainability', *Journal of Medicine and Philosophy*, 33(3): 241–261.

BEUC (2007) *Put Health First*, BEUC Position on the future of medicines in Europe, Brussels: European Consumers' Organisation, Ref X/59/2007–23/10/2007.

Björkman, J. W. (2004) 'Health sector reforms: measures, muddles and mires', in A. Rosenbaum, J. Nemec and K. Tolo (eds) *Public Health Care Systems: Opportunities for Public Management Education in Central and Eastern Europe*, Bratislava: Network of Institutes & Schools of PubAdm in CEE.

Blair, T. (1996): *New Britain: My Vision of a Young Country*, London: Fourth Estate.

—— (2002) *The Courage of Our Convictions: Why Reform of the Public Services is the Route to Social Justice*, London: Fabian Society.

Blomgren, M. (2003) 'Ordering a profession: Swedish nurses encounter new public management reforms', *Financial Accountability and Management*, 19(1): 45–71.

Blomgren, M. and Sundén, E. (2008) 'Constructing a European healthcare market: the private healthcare company Capio and the strategic aspect of the drive for transparency', *Social Science and Medicine*, 67(10): 1512–1520.

Blomqvist, P. (2002) *Ideas and Policy Convergence: Health Care Reforms in the Netherlands and Sweden in the 1990s*, New York: Columbia University Press.

—— (2004) 'The choice revolution: privatization of Swedish welfare services in the 1990s', *Social Policy and Administration*, 38(2): 139–155.

—— (2007) 'The role of ideas in policy change: healthcare reform in Sweden and the

Netherlands in the 1990s', Paper presented in the International Sociological Association RC19 conference, 5–8 September 2007.

Blomqvist, P. and Rothstein, B. (2000) *Välfärdstatens nya ansikte. Demokrati och marknadsreformer inom den offentliga sektorn*, Stockholm: Agora.

Bloomfield, B. P. and Danieli, A. (1995) 'The role of management consultants in the development of information technology: the indissoluble nature of socio-political and technical skills', *Journal of Management Studies*, 32(1): 23–46.

Bodenheimer, T., Lorig, K, Holman, H. and Grumbach, K. (2002) 'Patient self-management of chronic disease in primary care', *Journal of the American Medical Association*, 288 (19): 2469–2475.

Buchan, J. (2006) 'Migration of health workers in Europe: a policy problem or policy solution?', in C-A. Dubois, E. Nolte and M. McKee (eds) *Human Resources for Health in Europe*, Maidenhead: Open University Press.

Buchan, J. and Sochalski, J. (2004) 'The migration of nurses: trends and policies', *Bulletin of World Health Organisation*, 82(8): 587–594.

Burns, D., Hambleton, R. and Hogget, P. (1994) *The Politics of Decentralisation: Revitalising Local Democracy*, Basingstoke: Macmillan.

Cabiedes, L. and Guillen, A. (2001) 'Adopting and adapting managed competition: healthcare reform in Southern Europe', *Social Science and Medicine*, 52(8): 1205–1217.

Callaghan, G. and Wistow, G. (2006) 'Publics, patients, citizens, consumers? Power and decision making in primary healthcare', *Public Administration*, 84(3): 583–601.

Calman, K. and Hine, D. (1995) *A Policy Framework for Commissioning Cancer Services: A Report by the Expert Advisory Group on Cancer to the Chief Medical Officers of England and Wales*, London: Department of Health and the Welsh Office.

Calnan, M. and Gabe, J. (2001) 'From consumerism to partnership? Britain's National Health Service at the turn of the century', *International Journal of Health Services*, 31(1): 119–131.

Capio (2008) Capio website. History. European operations. http://www.capio.se/en/About-Capio/History/. (accessed 17 December 2008).

Carema (2008) 'Ägarstruktur', http://www.carema.se/huvudnavigation/omcarema/agare.4.5d31824f11d6cef7d74800025786.html (accessed 14 April 2009).

Carrol, E. (2004) 'International organisations and welfare states at odds? The case of Sweden', in K. Armingeon and M. Beyeler (eds) *The OECD and the European Welfare States*, Cheltenham: Edward Elgar.

Cayton, H. (2006) 'Patients as entrepreneurs: who is in charge of change?', in E. Andersson, J. Tritter and R. Wilson (eds) *Healthy Democracy: The Future of Involvement in Health and Social Care*, London: Involve and the NHS Centre for Involvement.

Chang, L., Garside, P., Wait, P. and Morris, Z. (2005) 'Environmental scan', in Z. Morris, L. Chang, S. Dawson and P. Garside (eds) *Policy Futures for UK Health*, Oxford: Radcliffe Publishing for the Nuffield Trust.

Chief Medical Officer (2006) *The Expert Patients Programme*, London: Department of Health.

Coen, D. (2007) *Lobbying in the European Union*, November 2007. PE 393.266. Directorate-General Internal Policies, Citizen rights and constitutional affairs, Paper requested by the European Parliaments Constitutional Committee.

Consumer Agency (2006) *Sosiaali- ja terveyspalveluiden asiakkaan oikeusasema terveyspalveluissa. Vertailu yksityisten ja kunnan järjestämien palveluiden välillä.* Kuluttajaviraston julkaisusarja 9/2006.

Coote, A. (2006) 'The role of citizens and service users in regulating healthcare', in E. Anderson, J. Tritter, and R. Wilson (eds) *Healthy Democracy: Involving People in Health and Social Care*, London: Involve.

Coulter, A. (2002) *The Autonomous Patient Ending Paternalism in Medical Care*, London: The Nuffield Trust.

—— (2006) 'Patient engagement: why is it so important?', in E. Andersson, J.Tritter and R. Wilson (eds) *Healthy Democracy*, London: Involve and NHS Centre for Involvement, pp. 27–35.

Coulter, A. and Magee, H. (2003) *The European Patient of the Future*, Berkshire: McGraw Hill and Open University Press.

Council of Europe (1980) *Recommendation No (80) 4 of the Committee of Ministers to the Member States Concerning the Patient as an Active Participant in His Own Treatment*, Strasbourg: Council of Europe.

—— (1986) *Recommendation No (86) 5 of the Committee of Ministers to the Member States on Making Medical Care Universally Available*, Strasbourg: Council of Europe.

—— (1996) *Fifth Conference of Health Ministers: Equity and Patient Rights in the Context of Health Care Reforms, 7–8 November, Warsaw, Poland*, http://www.coe.int/t/dg3/health/Conferences/1996SGreport_en.asp#P76_521 (accessed 14 April 2009).

—— (1997) 'Network for an Exchange of Information: A proposal of the 5th Conference of European Health ministers' (cdsp(97)10), Item 11.1, *Fifth Conference of Health Ministers: Equity and Patients' Rights in the context of health reforms, 7–8 November 1996, Warsaw, Poland*, Strasbourg: Council of Europe.

—— (2000) *Recommendation no. R(2000)5 of the Committee of Ministers to Member States on the Development of Structures for Citizen and Patient Participation in the Decision-making Process Affecting Health Care*, Including appendix on guidelines, Strasbourg: Council of Europe, https://wcd.coe.int/ViewDoc.jsp?id=340437&BackColorInternet=9999CC&BackColorIntranet=FF BB55&BackColorLogged=FFAC75 (accessed 14 April 2009).

Council of the European Union (2004) *The 2004 update of the Broad Guidelines of the Economic Policies of the Member States and the Community (for the 2003–2005 period) 10676/04*, Brussels: Council of the European Union.

Council of the European Union (2006) *Council Conclusions on Common Values and Principles in EU Health Systems*, 2733rd Employment, Social Policy, Health and Consumer Affairs Council Meeting, Luxembourg, 1–2 June.

Craig, D. (2006) *Plundering the Public Sector: How New Labour are Letting Consultants Run Off With £70 Billion of Our Money*, London: Constable & Robinson.

Croft, S. and Beresford, P. (1993) 'User involvement, citizenship and social policy', *Critical Social Policy*, 9(26): 5–18.

—— (1995) 'Whose empowerment? Equalising the competing discourses in community care', in R. Jack (ed.) *Empowerment in Community Care*, London: Chapman & Hall, pp. 59–73.

Dahl, R. (1961) *Who Governs?*, New Haven: Yale University Press.

Dahlgren, G. (1990) 'Strategies for health financing in Kenya – the difficult birth of a new policy', *Scandinavian Journal of Social Medicine*, 46 (supplement): 67–81.
—— (1994) *Framtidens sjukvårdmarknader. Vinnare och förlorare*, Stockholm: Natur och Kultur.
—— (2008) 'Neoliberal reforms in Swedish primary healthcare: for whom and for what purpose', *International Journal of Health Services*, 38(4): 697–715.
Dale, J., Sandhu, H., Lall, R. and Glucksman, E. (2008) 'The patient, the doctor and the emergency department: a cross-sectional stuffy of patient-centredness in 1990 and 2005', *Patient Education and Counselling*, 72(2): 320–329.
Davies, C., Wetherell, M. and Barnett, E. (2006) *Citizens at the Centre: Deliberative Participation in Healthcare Decisions*, Bristol: Policy Press.
Dawson, S. and Sausman, C. (2005) *Future Health Organisations and Systems*, Basingstoke: Palgrave Macmillan.
Daykin, N., Rimmer, J., Turton, P., Evans, S., Sanidas, M., Tritter, J. and Langton, H. (2002) 'Enhancing user involvement through interprofessional education in health-care: the case of cancer services', *Learning in Health and Social Care*, 1(3): 122–132.
Decision of the European Parliament and of the European Council (2006) 'Establishing for the period 2007 to 2013 the programme "Europe for citizens" to promote active European citizenship', *Official Journal of the European Union* L378/32, 27 December 2006.
Department of Communities and Local Government (2007) *Delivering Health and Well-being in Partnership: The Crucial Role of the New Local Performance Framework*, London: Department of Communities and Local Government.
Department of Health (1989) *Working for Patients* (CM 555), London: HMSO.
—— (1991) *The Patient's Charter*, London: The Stationery Office.
—— (1996) *Primary Care Delivering the Future* (Cm3512), London: Department of Health.
—— (1997) *The New NHS: Modern, Dependable* (Cm3807), London: Department of Health. See also <http://www.dh.gov.uk/en/Publicationsandstatistics/Publications/PublicationsPolicyAndGuidance/OH_4008869>.
—— (1999a) *Patient and Public Involvement in the New NHS*, London: Department of Health.
—— (1999b) *Saving Lives: Our Healthier Nation* (CM 4386), London: Department of Health.
—— (2000) *NHS Plan: A Plan for Investment, a Plan for Reform* (Cm 4818), London: Department of Health.
—— (2001a) *Shifting the Balance of Power within the NHS*, London: Department of Health.
—— (2001b) *The Report of the Public Inquiry into Children's Heart Surgery at the Bristol Royal Infirmary 1984–1995: Learning from Bristol* (Cm5207(I)), London: Department of Health.
—— (2002) *Reforming NHS Financial Flows: Introducing Payment by Results*, London: Department of Health.
—— (2003a) *Building on the Best: Choice, Responsiveness and Equity in the NHS (Cm 6268)*, London: Department of Health.
—— (2003b) *Strengthening Accountability: Involving Patients and the Public. Practice Guidance – Section 11 of the Health and Social Care Act 2001*, London: Department of Health.

—— (2003c) *Choice, Responsiveness and Equity in the NHS and Social Care: A National Consultation*, London: Department of Health.

—— (2004a) *The NHS Improvement Plan: Putting People at the Heart of Public Services* (Cm 6268), London: Department of Health.

—— (2004b) *Choosing Health: Making Healthy Choices Easier* (Cm 6374), London: Department of Health.

—— (2004c) *National Standards, Local Action: Health and Social Care – Standards and Planning Framework 2005/06–2007/08* (Cm 6374), London: Department of Health.

—— (2005a) *Creating a Patient-Led NHS: Delivering the NHS Improvement Plan*, London: Department of Health.

—— (2005b) *Commissioning a Patient-Led NHS* (Cm 6268), London: Department of Health.

—— (2006a) *Concluding the Review of Patient and Public Involvement – Recommendations to Ministers from the Expert Panel*, London: Department of Health.

—— (2006b) *A Stronger Local Voice: A Framework for Creating a Stronger Local Voice in the Development of Health and Social Care Services*, London: Department of Health.

—— (2006c) *Choice Matters: Increasing Choice Improves Patients' Experiences*, London: Department of Health.

—— (2006d) *Health Reform in England: Update and Commissioning Framework*, London: Department of Health.

—— (2007) *World Class Commissioning: Vision*, London: Department of Health.

—— (2008a) *Real Involvement: Working with People to Improve Health Services*, London: Department of Health.

—— (2008b) *Framework for Procuring External Support for Commissioners*, London: Department of Health.

—— (2008c) *A Consultation on the NHS Constitution*, London: Department of Health.

—— (2008d) *Real Involvement: Working with People to Improve Health Services*, London: Department of Health.

Department of Health and NHS Executive (1996) *Patient Partnership: Building a Collaborative Strategy*, London: Department of Health.

Diallo, K. (2004) 'Data on the migration of health-care workers: sources, uses and challenges', *Bulletin of the World Health Organisation*, 82(8): 601–607.

Dixon, A., Le Grand, J. Henderson, J., Murray, R. and Poteliakhoff, E. (2003) 'Is the NHS equitable? A review of the evidence', *LSE Health and Social Care Discussion Paper Number 11*, London: London School of Economics.

Docteur, E. and Oxley, H. (2003) *Health Care Systems: Lessons from the Reform Experience*, Paris: OECD/ELSA/WD/HEA.

Docteur, E., Suppanz, H. and Woo, J. (2003) 'The US health system: an assessment and prospective directions for reform', *Working Paper of the Economic Department of the OECD* (no. 350), Paris: OECD.

Donaldson, L. (2001) 'Patients to become the key decision-makers in their own care', Department of Health Press Release 14 September, http://www.dh.gov. uk/en/ Publicationsandstatistics/Pressreleases/DH_4010913 (accessed 12 April 2009).

—— (2008) 'The future of healthcare: improving patient safety, access to healthcare, patient information and patient involvement', *3rd Global Patients Congress*, Budapest, Hungary, 21 February.

Doran, E. and Henry, D. A. (2008) 'Australian pharmaceutical policy: price control, equity, and drug innovation in Australia', *Journal of Public Health Policy*, 29(1): 106–120.

Drache, D. and Sullivan, T. (eds) (1999) *Health Reform: Public Success and Private Failure*, London: Routledge.

Dredge, R. and Capaldi, A. (2005) 'Dealing with unavoidable input cost differences in health and local government', *University of Warwick Health Services Partnership Discussion Paper Eight*, Coventry: Institute of Governance and Public Management.

Eduskunta (2008) *Työelämä- ja tasa-arvolautakunnan lausunto* TyVL 13/2008–U58/2004. http://www.eduskunta.fi/faktatmp/utatmp/akxtmp/tyvl_13_2008_p.shtml (accessed 16 December 2008).

eGov Monitor (2006) 'Patient mobility: commission to launch public consultation on EU framework for health services', *eGov Monitor* 7.09.06 http://www.egovmonitor.com/node/7479/print (accessed 25 February 2008).

Ekonomikomission (1993) *Nya villkor för ekonomi och politik, Statens offentliga utredningar*, Stockholm: Allmänna förlaget.

Englund, P. (1999) 'Swedish banking crisis: roots and consequences', *Oxford Review of Economic Policy*, 15(3): 80–97.

Enthoven, A. (1980) *Health Plan: The Only Practical Solution to the Soaring Cost of Medical Care*, Reading, MA: Addison-Wesley.

—— (1985) *Reflections on the Management of the National Health Service*, London: Nuffield Provincial Hospitals' Trust.

—— (1989) 'What can Europeans learn from Americans about financing and organization of medical care?', *Health Care Financing Review*, Annual Supplement: 49–63.

—— (1993) 'The history and principles of managed competition', *Health Affairs*, 12(Supplement): 24–48.

—— (2002) 'Introducing market forces into healthcare: a tale of two countries', Presented at the *Fourth European Conference on Health Economics*, Paris, July 10.

Eronen, A., Londen, P., Perälahti, A., Siltaniemi, A. and Särkelä, R. (2006) *Sosiaalibarometri. Sosiaali- ja terveysturvan*, Helsinki: Sosiaali- ja terveysturvan keskusliitto.

European Centre for Health Policy and WHO Regional Officer for Europe (1999) *Gothenburg Consensus Paper: Health Impact Assessment, Main Concepts and Suggested Approach*, Copenhagen: WHO Regional Office for Europe.

European Charter (2000) 'Charter of Fundamental Rights of the European Union', *Official Journal of the European Union*, 2000/C 364/01.

European Commission (2001) *White Paper: European Governance*, COM (2001) 428 final, Brussels: European Commission.

—— (2003) *Green Paper on Services of General Interest*, COM (2003) 270 final, Brussels: European Commission.

—— (2004a) *Directive on Services on the Internal Market*, COM 2004 2 final/3, Brussels: European Commission.

—— (2004b) *Modernising Social Protection for the Development of High-Quality, Accessible and Sustainable Health Care and Long-Term Care: Support for the National Strategies Using the 'Open Method of Coordination'*, COM (2004) 304 final, Brussels: European Commission.

—— (2004c) *White Paper on Services of General Interest*, COM (2004) 374 final, Brussels: European Commission.

—— (2004d) *e-Health – Making Healthcare Better for European Citizens: An Action*

Plan for a European e-Health Area, COM (2004) 356, Brussels: European Commission.

—— (2004e) *European Competitiveness Report 2004*, SEC (2004) 1397 Staff Working Paper, Brussels: European Commission.

—— (2006a) *Amended Proposal for a Decision of the European Parliament and Council, Establishing a Second Programme of Community Action in the Field of Health (2007–2013) (COM (2006) 234 Final)*, Brussels: Commission of the European Community.

—— (2006b) *Consultation Regarding Community Action on Health Services*, SEC (2006) 1195/4, Brussels: European Commission.

—— (2006c) *Commission Interpretative Communication on the Community Law Applicable to Contract Awards Not or Not Fully Subject to the Provisions of the Public Procurement Directives*, 2006/C 179/02, Brussels: European Commission.

—— (2006d) *Citizens' Agenda: Delivering Results for Europe*, COM (2006) 211 final, Brussels: European Commission.

—— (2007a) *Together for Health*, White Paper, A strategic approach for the European Union 2008–2013 COM (2007)630 final, Brussels: European Commission.

—— (2007b) *Communication from the European Commission Accompanying the Communication on 'a Single Market for 21st Century Europe' Services of General Interest, Including Social Services of General Interest: A New European Commitment*, COM 2007 (724 final); SEC 2007 (1514); SEC 2007 (1515); SEC 2007, (1516), Brussels: European Commission.

—— (2007c) *A Single Market for the 21st Century*, COM (2007) 724 final, Brussels: European Commission.

—— (2008a) Proposal for a *Directive of the European Parliament and of the Council on the Application of Patient's Rights in Cross-border Healthcare*, COM (2008) 414 final, Brussels: European Commission.

—— (2008b) *Pharmaceutical Sector Inquiry*, Preliminary Report, DG Competition Staff Working Paper, Executive Summary, Brussels: European Commission.

—— (2008c) *Safe, Innovative and Accessible Medicines: A Renewed Vision for the Pharmaceutical Sector*, COM (2008) 666, Brussels: European Commission.

—— (2008d) *Recommendation on Cross-Border Interoperability of Electronic Health Record Systems*, COM (2008) 3282 final, Brussels: European Commission.

European Court of Justice (ECJ) (1998a) *Judgement of the Court Case C-120/95 Nicolas Decker vs Caisse de Maladie des Employees Prives*, 28 April 1998.

—— (1998b) *Judgment of the Court Case C-158/96 Raymond Kohll vs Union des Caisses de Maladie*, 28 April 1998.

—— (2000) *Judgment of the Court Case C-303/98 Sindicato de Medicos Asistencia Publica (SIMAP) vs Conselleria de Sanidad y Consumo de la Generlidad Valenciana*, 3 October 2000.

—— (2003) *Judgment of the Court Case C-151/02 Landeshauptstadt Kiel vs Norbert Jaeger*, 9 September 2003.

—— (2005a) *Judgment of the Court Case C-231/03 Consorzio Aziende Metano (Coname) vs Comune de Cingia* de' Botti, 21 July 2005.

—— (2005b) *Opinion of Advocate General of the Court Case C-231/03Consorzio Aziende Metano (Coname) vs Comune de Cingia de' Botti*, 12 April 2005.

—— (2006) *Judgment of the Court Case C-372/04 The Queen, on the Application of Yvonne Watts vs Bedford Primary Care Trust and Secretary of State for Health*, 16 May 2006.

European Health Management Association (2000) *The Impact of Market Forces on Health Systems: A Review of Evidence in the 15 European Member States*, Brussels: European Health Management Association.

European Parliament (2008a) *Draft Report on the Application of Patient Rights in Cross-Border Health Care*, Rapporteur John Bowis, Brussels: European Parliament.

—— (2008b) *Report on the Framework for the Activities of Interest Representatives (lobbyists) in the European Union*, Rapporteur: Alexander Stubb, Constitutional Affairs Committee, Brussels: European Parliament.

—— (2008c) *Framework for the Activities of Lobbyists in the European Union Institutions*, Brussels: European Parliament.

European Union (2002) *Decision of the Council and European Parliament 23 September 2002 Adopting a Programme of Community Action in the Field of Public Health (2003–2008) (1786/2002/EC)*, Brussels: European Union.

—— (2005) *Council Decision of 17 Feb 2005 on the Conclusion, on Behalf of the EC of the Convention on Access to Information, Public Participation in Decision-Making and Access to Justice in Environmental Matters (2005/370/EC)*, Brussels: European Union.

Evans, R.G. (2005) 'Fellow travellers on a contested path: power, purpose, and the evolution of European healthcare systems', *Journal of Health Politics, Policy and Law*, 30(1–2): 277–293.

Exworthy, M. and Peckham, S. (2006) 'Access, choice and travel: implication for health policy', *Social Policy and Administration*, 40(3): 267–287.

Fallberg, L. (2000) 'Patient rights in the Nordic countries', *European Journal of Health Law*, 7(2): 123–143.

Famna (2008) What Famna does. (accessed 15 December 2008).

Farrell, C. (2004) *Patient and Public Involvement in Health: The Evidence for Policy Implementation*, London: Department of Health.

Feldberg, G. and Vipond, R. (1999) 'The virus of consumerism', in Drache and Sullivan (1999), pp. 448–464.

Fidler, D. (2003) 'Legal review of the General Agreement on Trade in Services (GATS) from a health policy perspective', *Globalisation, Trade and Health Working Paper Series*, Geneva: World Health Organisation

Fidler, D. and Drager, N. (2004) *GATS and Health-Related Services: Managing Liberalization of Trade in Services from a Health Policy Perspective*, Geneva: World Health Organization.

Fieldhouse, E., Tranmer, M. and Russell, A. (2007) 'Something about young people or something about elections? Electoral participation of young people in Europe: Evidence from a multilevel analysis of the European Social Survey', *European Journal of Political Research*, 46(6): 797–822.

Fielding, S. (2003) *The Labour Party: Continuity and Change in the Making of 'New Labour'*, Basingstoke: Palgrave.

Final Text (1996) *Final Text approved in the Fifth Conference of Health Ministers on Equity and Patients' rights in the Context of Health Reforms*, 7–8 November 1996, Warsaw, Poland.

Finlay, I. and Crisp, N. (2008) 'Drugs for cancer and copayments', *British Medical Journal*, 337(7660): a527.

Finnish Constitution (1999) *Constitution of Finland*, 11 June 1999, 731/1999.

Florin, D. and Dixon, J. (2004) 'Public involvement in healthcare', *British Medical Journal*, 328(7432): 159–161.

Forma P, Kuivalainen S, Niemelä M, Saarinen A (2007a) *Kuinka hyvinvointivaltio kesytetään?* Turun Yliopiston Sosiaalipolitiikan laitoksen julkaisuja 2007: B32, Turku: TurunYliopisto.

Forma P, Kallio J, Pirttilä J, Uusitalo R (2007b) *Kuinka hyvinvointivaltio pelastetaan*, Kelan tutkimusosasto, Sosiaali- ja terveysturvan tutkimuksia 89, Helsinki: Kansanelakelaitas.

Försäkringskassan (2007) *Gränsövreskridande vård inom EU/EES*. Försäkringskassan svar på regeringsuppdrag, Stockholm: Försäkringskassan.

Fotaki, M. (2007) 'Patient choice in healthcare in England and Sweden: from quasi-market and back to market? A comparative analysis of failure in unlearning', *Public Administration*, 85 (4): 1059–1075.

Franklin, M. (2004) *Voter Turnout and the Dynamics of Elector Competition in Established Democracies since 1945*, Cambridge: Cambridge University Press.

Fredman, S. (2006) 'Transformation or dilution: fundamental rights in the EU social space', *European Law Journal*, 12(1): 41–60.

Fredriskson, S. and Martikainen, T. (eds)(2006) *Kilpailuttamisen kokemukset*, Kunnallisalan kehittämissäätiö, Vammala: Vammalan kirjapaino.

Fredriksson, M. and Winblad, U. (2008) 'Consequences of a decentralised healthcare governance model: measuring regional authority support for patient choice in Sweden', *Social Science and Medicine*, 67(2): 271–279.

Freeman, R. (1998) 'Competition in context: the politics of healthcare reform in Europe', *International Journal for Quality in Health Care*, 10(5): 395–401.

Garpenby, P. (1992) 'The transformation of the Swedish healthcare system, or the hasty rejection of the rational planning model', *Journal of European Social Policy*, 2(1): 17–31.

Glenngård, A. H., Hjalte, F., Svensson, M., Anell, A. and Bankauskaite, V. (2005) *Health Systems in Transition: Sweden*, Copenhagen: WHO Regional Office for Europe on behalf of the European Observatory on Health Systems and Policies.

Goes, E. (2004) 'The Third Way and the politics of community', in S. Hale, W. Leggett and L. Martell (eds) *The Third Way and Beyond: Criticisms, Futures, Alternatives*, Manchester: Manchester University Press.

Goroya, A. and Scambler, G. (1998) 'From the old to New Public Health: role tensions and contradictions', *Critical Public Health*, 8(2): 141–151.

Gott, M., Stevens, T., Small, N. and Ahmedzai, H. (2002) 'Involving users, improving services: the example of cancer', *British Journal of Clinical Governance*, 7(2): 81–85.

Government of Western Australia (2006) *Working Together: Involving Community and Stakeholder in Decision-Making*, Perth: Department of the Premier and Cabinet.

Gramberger, M. (2001) *Citizens as Partners: OECD Handbook on Information, Consultation and Public Participation in Policy Making*, Paris: OECD.

Greener, I. (2003) 'Who choosing what? The evolution of the word "choice" in the NHS and its implications for New Labour', *Social Policy Review*, 15: 49–67.

Green-Pedersen, C. (2002) 'New Public Management reforms of the Danish and Swedish welfare states: the role of different social democratic responses', *Governance*, 15(2): 271–294.

Greenwood, J. (1997) *Representing Interests in the European Union*, Basingstoke: Macmillan.

Grieshaber-Otto, R. and Sinclair, S. (2004) *Bad Medicine: Trade Treaties, Privatisation and Health Care Reforms in Canada*, Ottawa: Canada Centre for Policy Alternatives.

Griffiths, R. (1983) *NHS Management Inquiry Report*, London: Department of Health and Social Security.

Haas, E. B. (1958) *The Uniting of Europe*, London: Stevens.

Haavisto, I., Kiljunen, P. and Nuberg, M. (2007) *Satavuotias kuntotestissä*, EVA:n kansallinen arvo- ja asennetutkimus 2007, http://www.eva.fi (accessed 12 December 2008).

Häkkinen, U. (1987) 'Terveydenhuollon talous sekä julkisen ja yksityisen sektorin suhde Suomessa ja muissa OECD maissa', *Sosiaalilääketieteellinen Aikakauslehti*, 24(2): 93–104.

Hallas, J. (1976) *CHCs in Action*, London: Nuffield Provincial Hospitals Trust.

Ham, C. (1999) *Health Policy in Britain: Public Policy and Politics*, Basingstoke: Palgrave.

Ham, C. and Brommels, M. (1994) 'Healthcare reforms in the Netherlands, Sweden and the United Kingdom', *Health Affairs*, 13(5): 106–119.

Hamblin, R. (1998) 'Trusts', in J. Le Grand, N. Mays and J. A. Mulligan (eds) *Learning from the NHS Internal Market: A Review of the Evidence*, London: King's Fund.

Harrison, M. (2004) *Implementing Change in Health Systems: Market reforms in the United Kingdom, Sweden & the Netherlands*, London: Sage.

Harrison, M. I. and Calltorp, J. (2000) 'The reorientation of market-oriented reforms in Swedish healthcare', *Health Policy*, 50(3): 219–240.

Harrison, S. and Mort, M. (1998) 'Which champions, which people? Public and user involvement in healthcare as a technology of legitimation', *Social Policy & Administrations*, 32: 60–70.

Haverinen R (1999) *Palvelusitoumukset ja hyvinvointivaltion käänne*,Tutkimuksia, Helsinki: STAKES.

Hayek, F. A. (1979) *Law, Legislation, and Liberty, Vol. 3: The Political Order of a Free People*, London: Routledge & Kegan Paul.

Health Action International (HAI) (2005) *Does the European Patients' Forum Represent Patient or Industry Interests? A Case Study in the Need for Mandatory Financial Disclosure*, Amsterdam: Health Action International.

Health Canada (2000) *Policy Toolkit for Public Involvement in Decision Making*, Ottawa: Minister of Public Works and Government Services Canada.

Health Committee (1995) *1st Report 1994/95, Priority Setting in the NHS*, London: HMSO.

Heikkilä, M., Kautto, M. and Teperi, J. (2005) *Julkinen hyvinvointivastuu sosiaali- ja terveydenhuollossa*. Valtioneuvoston kanslian julkaisusarja 5/2005.

Held, D., McGrew, A., Goldblatt, D. and Perraton, J. (1999) *Global Transformations: Politics, Economics and Culture*, Cambridge: Polity Press.

Henderson, S. and Petersen, A. (eds) (2002) *Consuming Health: The Commodification of Health Care*, London and New York: Routledge.

Henke, K.-D. and Schreyögg, J. (2004) *Towards Sustainable Health Care Systems: Strategies in France, Germany, Japan and the Netherlands: A Comparative Study*, Berlin: International Social Security Association.

Her Majesty's Treasury (2003) *PFI: Meeting the Investment Challenge*, London: HM Treasury.

Hervey, T. (2006) 'The right to health in EU law,' in T. Hervey and J. Kenner (2006).

Hervey, T. and Kenner, J. (eds) (2006) *Economic and Social Rights Under the EU Charter of Fundamental Rights: A Legal Perspective*, Oxford: Hart Publishing.

Herxheimer, A. (2003) 'Relationship between the pharmaceutical industry and patients' organisations', *British Medical Journal*, 326(7400): 1208–1210.

High Level Committee (2001) *The Internal Market and Health Services*, 17.12.2001, Brussels: European Commission.

Hirschman, A. (1970) *Exit, Voice and Loyalty: Responses to Decline in Firms, Organizations and States*, London: Harvard University Press.

Hodge, G. and Bowman, D. (2006) 'The "consultocracy": the business of reforming government", in G. Hodge (ed.) *Privatization and Market Development: Global Movements in Public Policy Ideas*, Cheltenham: Edward Elgar, pp. 97–126.

Hogg, C. (2008) *Citizens, Consumers and the NHS: Capturing Voices*, London: Palgrave Macmillan.

Holland, W. and Fotaki, M. (2006) 'Choice in healthcare: old wine in new bottles?', *Eurohealth*, 12(2): 1–3.

Hood, C. (1991) 'A public management for all seasons?', *Public Administration*, 69(1): 3–9.

Hunt, P. (2007) 'Remarks to the Press', Visit to Sweden of Professor Paul Hunt, UN Special Rapporteur on the right to the highest attainable standard of health, 18 June 2007, Stockholm, http://74.125.77.132/search?q=cache:wrIOrQ4dyUIJ:www2.essex.ac.uk/human_rights_centre/rth/docs/oral%2520remarks%2520to%2520press%2520monday%252018%2520june%25202007.doc+18+june+2007+Professor+Paul+Hunt+Sweden+is+integrating+human+rights&cd=6&hl=en&ct=clnk (accessed 15 April 2009).

Ignatieff, M. (1995) 'The myth of citizenship', in R. Beiner (ed.) *Theorising Citizenship*, Albany: SUNY Press.

International Alliance of Patients' Organizations (IAPO) (2005) IAPO policy statement on patient involvement', http://www.patientsorganizations.org/showarticle.pl?id=283&n=3102 (accessed 19 July 2008).

—— (2006) 'Declaration on patient-centred healthcare', http://www.patientsorganizations.org/showarticle.pl?id=283&n=3102 (accessed 19 July 2008).

Involve (2003) 'Strategic Plan 2003–2006: Creating the Expert Resource', Involve: Eastleigh Hampshire, http://www.invo.org.uk/pdfs/involve%20strategic%20plan%202003.pdf (accessed 17 December 2008).

Järvelin, J. (2002) *Health Care Systems in Transition: Finland*, Brussels: European Observatory on Health Care Systems.

Joerges, C., Meny, Y., Weiler, J. H. H. (eds) (2001) Mountain or molehill? A critical appraisal of the commission White Paper on governance', http://www.jeanmonnet-program.org/papers/01/010601.html (accessed 15 December 2008).

Johansson, K. (2005) *Motion till riksdagen*, 2005/06sk526.

Jordan, J., Dowswell, T., Harrison, S., Lilford, R. and Mort, M. (1998) 'Health needs assessment: whose priorities? Listening to users and the public', *British Medical Journal*, 316: 16681–670.

Kallio, J. (2007) 'Kansalaisten asennoituminen kunnallisten palveluiden markkinoistumiseen vuosina 1996–2004', *Yhteiskuntapolitiikka*, 72(3): 239–255.

Kanniainen V (2002) *Puhtia Hyvinvointiyhteiskunnan Purjeisiin, Peruspalveluja uudella tavalla*, Helsinki: EVA.

Kauppa-ja teollisuusministeriö (2001) *Laatua ja tehokkuutta palvelujen kilpailulla*. Kauppa- ja teollisuusministeriön työryhmä ja toimikuntarapotteja 17: 2001, Helsinki: Elinkeino-osasto.

—— (2007) *Julkisesti rahoitettujen sosiaali- ja terveyspalvelujen kaupallistaminen ja vienti osana suomalaisen hyvinvointiklusterin vienninedistämistä*, KTM Julkaisuja: 25.

Kauppakamari (2008) Helsingin Seudun kauppakamari, Julkiset palvelumarkkinat toimimaan – projekti, Available from: http://www.espoonkauppakamari.fi/index.phtml?s=275 (accessed 15 December 2008).

Kauppinen, S. and Niskanen, T. (2005) *Yksityinen palvelutuotanto sosiaali- ja terveyshuollossa*, Helsinki: STAKES.

Keep our NHS Public (2009) http://www.keepournhspublic.com/index.php (accessed 12 April 2009).

Keskimäki, I. (2003) 'How did Finland's economic recession in the early 1990s affect socio-economic equity in the use of hospital care', *Social Science and Medicine*, 56(7): 1517–1530.

Kettl, D. F. (2000) 'Public administration at the millennium: the state of the field', *Journal of Public Administration Research and Theory*, 10(1): 7–34.

Kilpailuvirasto (1996) *Lausunto kilpailun esteistä terveyssektorilla*, Helsinki: Kilpailuvirasto.

—— (2001) *Markkinat ja kilpailu kuntien tuotantotoiminnassa*, Helsinki: Kilpailuvirasto, Selvityksiä 1/2001.

—— (2006) Yrityskaupan hyväksyminen H-Careholding AB/Mehiläinen Oyj, Dnro 253/81/2006. 3. May 2006, http://www.kilpailuvirasto.fi/cgi-bin/suomi.cgi?sivu=ratk/r-2006–81–0253 (accessed 14 April 2009).

Klein, R. (2001) *The New Politics of the NHS*, 4th ed., Harlow: Pearson.

Klein, R. and Lewis, J. (1976) *The Politics of Consumer Representation: A Study of Community Health Councils*, London: Centre for Studies in Social Policy.

Koivusalo, M. (2001) *Terveyspalveluiden kilpailuttaminen. Kilpailuttamisraportti*, Helsinki: STAKES.

—— (2003a) 'Health systems, solidarity and other European policies', in K. Sen (ed.) *Restructuring Health Services: Changing Contexts and Comparative Perspectives*, London: Zed Books.

—— (2003b) 'Assessing health policy implications of WTO trade and investment agreements', in K. Lee (ed.) *Health Impacts of Globalisation: Towards Global Governance*, Basingstoke: Palgrave.

Koivusalo, M. and Ollila, E. (1997) *Making a Healthy World: Agencies, Actors and Policies in International Health*, London: Zed Books.

Koivusalo, M. and Tritter, J. (2006) 'The Globalisation of Health Care Reforms: The Impact and Response to Commercialisation in Different National Contexts', *16th International Sociological Association World Congress of Sociology*, Durban, South Africa, 23–29 July.

Koivusalo, M., Santana, P. and Wyss, K. (2007) 'Equity aspects of decentralisation and re-centralisation', in R. Saltman, V. Bankauskaite and K. Vrangbæk (eds) *Decentralisation in Health Care: Strategies and Outcomes*, Maidenhead: WHO Observatory and Open University Press.

Koivusalo, M., Schrecker, T. and Labonte, R. (2009) 'Globalisation and national policy space for health', in R. Labonte, T. Schrecker, V. Runner and C. Packer (eds) *Globalization and Health*, London: Routledge.

Konkurrensverkett (2008) *Yttrande, Lov att välja – lag om valfrihetssystem*, 19.05.2005. Dnr 185/2008.

Korkman, S., Lassila, J., Määttä, R. and Valkonen, T. (2007) *Hyvinvointivaltion rahoitus- riittävätkö rahat, kuka maksaa? ETLA*, Helsinki: Yliopistopaino.

Krajewski, M. (2003) 'Public services and trade liberalization: mapping the legal framework', *Journal of International Economic Law*, 6(2): 341–367.

Kuntaliitto (2008) Kunta- ja palvelurakenneuudistus etenee suunnitelmista toteutukseen, http://www.kunnat.net/k_peruslistasivu.asp?path=1;55264;55275;82183; 127674;126210;128227;128228 (accessed 15 December 2008).

Lääketeollisuus (2008) Mitä Norja edellä sitä Suomi perässä, Tiedote, 07.05.2008 Press Release, *What Norway does first, Finland will follow*, http://www.laaketeollisuus.fi/page.php?page_id=99&offset=0&news_id=289 (accessed 15 December 2008).

Lähdesmäki, K. (2003) 'New public management ju julkisen sektorin uudistaminen', *Acto Wasaensia*, No. 113, Hallintotiede 7, Universitas Wasaensis.

Lammy, D. (2002) 'New era in patient and public involvement in NHS', London: Department of Health, http://nds.coi.gov.uk/environment/fullDetail.asp?Release ID=31025&NewsAreaID=2&NavigatedFromDepartment=False (accessed on 12 April 2009).

Lapsley, I. and Oldfield, R. (2001) 'Transforming the public sector: management consultants as agents of change', *The European Accounting Review*,10(3): 523–543.

Larsson, D., Uberbacher, O. and Johansson, C. (2004) 'EU-anpassad arbetstid kräver inte fler läkare', *Läkartidningen*, 101(24): 2126.

Lee, K. and Goodman, H. (2002) 'Global policy networks: the propagation of healthcare financing reform since the 1980s,' in K. Lee, K. Buse and S. Fustukian (eds) *Health Policy in a Globalising World*, Cambridge: Cambridge University Press.

Leenen, H., Gevers, S. and Pinet, G. (2003) *The Rights of Patients in Europe: A Comparative Study*, Boston and Deventer: Kluwer Law and Taxation Publishers.

Le Grand, J. (2007) *The Other Invisible Hand: Delivering Public Services through Choice and Competition*, Princeton, NJ: Princeton University Press.

Le Grand J. and Bartlett, W. (1993) *Quasi-Markets and Social Policy*, Basingstoke: Macmillan.

Lethbridge, J. (2005) 'Strategies of multinational healthcare companies in Europe and Asia', in M. Mackintosh and M. Koivusalo (eds) *Commercialisation of Health Care: Global and Local Dynamics and Policy Responses*, Basingstoke: Palgrave.

Lewis, R. (2005a) 'The Sound of Silence', *Public Finance*, 13–19 May: 20–23.

—— (2005b) *Governing Foundation Trusts: A New Era for Public Accountability*, London: King's Fund.

Leydon, G, Boulton, M., Moynihan, C., Jones, A., Mossman, J., Boudioni, M. and McPherson, K. (2000) 'Cancer patients' information needs and information seeking behaviour: in depth interview study', *British Medical Journal*, 320(7239): 909–913.

Lindgren, B. and Roos, P. (1985) *Produktions, kostnads och produktivitetsutveckling inom offentligt bedriven hälso- och sjukvård 1960–1980*, Stockholm: Allmänna förlaget.

Lister, J. (2005) *Health Policy Reform: Driving the Wrong Way?*, London: Middlesex University Press.

Lith, P. (2001) *Julkisen sektorin palvelut ja palveluntuottajien kilpailutilanne*, Helsinki: Kauppa- ja teollisuusministeriö.

Lith, Pekka (2006) *Yritystoiminta ja kuntien ostopalvelut sosiaali- ja terveydenhuollossa*, Helsinki: Kauppa- ja teollisuusministeriö.

Lloyd, P. and Cummins, J. (2003) *Signposts Two: Putting Public and Patient Involvement into Practice*, London and Cardiff: OPM and Welsh Assembly Government.

London Ambulance Service (2004) *Patient and Public Involvement (PPI) – The LAS Approach*, http://www.londonambulance.nhs.uk/talkingtous/ppi/media/PPIstrategy.pdf (accessed 5 July 2008).

Lowson, K., West, P. Chaplin, S. and O'Reilly, D. (2002) *Evaluation of Patients Travelling Overseas: Final Report*, York: YHEC.

Luff, D. (2003) 'Regulation of health services and international trade law', in A. Mattoo and P. Sauve (eds) *Domestic Regulation and Service Trade Liberalisation*, New York: World Bank and Oxford University Press.

Lyon T. P. and Maxwell, J. W. (2004) 'Astroturf: interest group lobbying and corporate strategy', *Journal of Economics & Management Strategy*, 13(4): 561–597.

Mackintosh, M. and Koivusalo, M. (2005) 'Health systems and commercialisation: in search of good sense', in M. Mackintosh and M. Koivusalo (eds) *Commercialisation of Health Care: Global and Local Dynamics and Policy Responses*, Basingstoke: Palgrave.

Mahony, H. (2008) 'EU health bill pulled amid national and MEP criticism', euobserver. com 10 January, http://euobserver.com/?aid=25426 (accessed 14 April 2009).

Mandelson, P. (2007) 'Compulsory licensing of pharmaceutical patents in Thailand,' 10 July 2007, Brussels, http://www.actupparis.org/IMG/pdf/Letter_from_Mandelson_to_Thailand.pdf (accessed 14 April 2009).

Marinker, M. (ed.) (1996) *Sense & Sensibility in Healthcare*, London: BMJ Publishing Group.

Marquand, D. (2004) *Decline of the Public: The Hollowing Out of Citizenship*, Oxford: Polity Press.

Mattoo, A. and Wunsch, S. (2004) 'Pre-empting protectionism in services: the GATS and outsourcing', *Journal of International Economic Law*, 7(4): 765–800.

Mattoo, A. and Rathindran, R. (2006) 'How health insurance inhibits trade in healthcare', *Health Affairs*, 25(2): 358–368.

Maynard, A. (1993) 'Competition in the UK National Health Services: mission impossible?', *Health Policy*, 23(3):193–204.

Maynard, A. and Bloor, K. (1995) 'Healthcare reform: informing difficult choices', *International Journal of Health Planning and Management*, 10(3): 247–64.

Mehiläinen (2005) Osavuosikatsaus 1.1.–30.6.2005, Helsinki: Mehiläinen, http://www.mehilainen.fi/dyn/news/Osavuosikatsaus_Mehilainen_H105_290805.pdf (accessed 14 April 2009).

—— (2008) 'Corporate information', http://www.mehiläinen.fi/dynamic/fin7index.php?module=LangCompanyInfo (accessed 12 December 2008).

Mensah, K. (2005) 'International migration of healthcare staff: extent and policy responses, with illustrations from Ghana', in M. Mackintosh and M. Koivusalo (eds) *Commercialisation of Health Care: Global and Local Dynamics and Policy Responses*, Basingstoke: Palgrave.

Milburn, A. (2002) 'Statement by the Rt Hon Alan Milburn MP, Secretary of State for Health to the House of Commons about delivering the NHS Plan', London: Department of Health, http://www.dh.gov.uk/en/News/Speeches/Speecheslist/DH_4000795 (accessed on 12 April 2009).

—— (2003) 'Choices for All, address to NHS Chief Executives', 11 February, http://www.dh.gov.uk/en/News/Speeches/SpeechesList/DH_4000782 (accessed 12 April 2009).

Milewa, T., Harrison, S., Ahmad, W. and Tovey, P. (2002) 'Citizens' participation in primary healthcare planning: innovative citizenship practice in empirical perspective', *Critical Public Health*, 12(1): 39–53.

Miliband, D. (2006) 'Choice and voice in personalised learning', in *Personalising Education: Schooling for Tomorrow*, Paris: Organisation for Economic Co-operation and Development, pp. 21–30.

Mills, A., Bennett, S. and Russell, S. (2001) *The Challenge of Health Sector Reform: What Must Governments Do?*, Basingstoke: Palgrave.

Ministry of Health Planning (2001) *A New Era for Patient-Centred Health Care: Building a Sustainable, Accountable Structure for Delivery of High-Quality Patient Services*, British Columbia: Ministry of Health Planning.

Moore, M. (1995) *Creating Public Value: Strategic Management in Government*, Boston: Harvard University Press.

Moran, M. and Wood, B. (1996) 'The globalisation of healthcare policy?', in P. Gummett (ed.) *Globalisation and Public Policy*, London: Edward Elgar, pp. 125–142.

Morrell, K. (2006) 'Policy as narrative: New Labour's reform of the National Health Service', *Public Administration*, 84(2): 367–385.

Morris, Z., Chang, L., Dawson, S. and Garside, P. (eds) (2005) *Policy Futures for UK Health*, Oxford: Radcliffe Publishing for the Nuffield Trust.

Möttönen, S. and Niemelä, J. (2005) *Kunta ja kolmas sektori*, Yhteistyön uudet muodot, Jyväskylä: PS-kustannus.

Muir Gray, J. A., and Rutter, H. (2002) *The Resourceful Patient*, Oxford: eRosetta Press.

Mulcahy, L. and Lloyd-Bostock, S. (1994) 'Managers as third party dispute handlers in complaints about hospitals', *Law and Policy*, 16 (2): 185–202.

Mulcahy, L. and Tritter, J. (1998) 'Pathways, pyramids and icebergs? Mapping the links between dissatisfaction and complaints', *Sociology of Health and Illness*, 20 (6): 825–847.

Narashiman, V., Brown H., Pablos-Mendez, A., Adams, O., Dussault, G., Elzinga, G., Nordstrom, A., Habte, D., Jacobs, M., Solimano, G., Sewankambo, N., Wibulpolprasert, S., Evans, T. and Chen, L. (2003) 'Responding to the global human resource crisis', *The Lancet* 363: 1469–1472.

National Consumer Council (2004) *Making Public Services Personal: A New Compact for Public Services*, London: National Consumer Council.

Nätverk för (2008) *Nätverk för Genemsam Välfärd*, http://www. gemensamval-fard.se/index.php?page_id=17 (accessed 17 December 2008).

New Local Government Network (2009) http://www.nlgn.org.uk/public/about-nlgn/ (accessed 12 February 2009).

NHS Centre for Involvement (2007) *Key Principles of Effective Patient and Public Involvement*, Coventry: NHS Centre for Involvement.

NHS Confederation and National Primary and Care Trust Development Programme (NatPaCT) (2003) *Briefing 9: Quality and Outcomes under the New GMS Contract*, London: NHS Confederation.

NHS Executive (NHSE) (1995) *Priorities and Planning Guidance for the NHS 1996/97*, Leeds: NHSE.

NHS Executive (1996) *Priorities and Planning Guidance for the NHS, 1997/98*, Leeds: NHSE.

NHS Management Executive (NHSME) (1992) *Local Voices: The Views of Local People in Purchasing for Health*, London: Department of Health.

NHS Quality Improvement Scotland (2003) *Patient Focus and Public Involvement*, Edinburgh: NHS Quality Improvement Scotland.

Niemelä, M. (2008) *Julkisen sektorin pitkä kaari Valtava- uudistuksesta Parashankkeeseen*, Helsinki: KELA, Sosiaali- ja terveysturvan tutkimuksia 102: 2008.

Nutek (2007a) *Värd och omsorg- en brancsh med till-växt potential. Nya Fakta och Statistik*, Framtidens näringsliv 2007: 1

—— (2007b) *Gränslös vård och omsorg. Nya Fakta och Statistik*. Framtidens näringsliv 2007: 4.

Nutek and Almega (2007) *Sjukvården – en tjänstebranch med effectiviseringspotential. Nya trender mot patientfokus och produktivitet*. Stockholm: Nutek.

O'Harrow, R. (2000) 'Grass roots seeded by drugmaker', *Washington Post*, September 12: A01.

Oikeus ja Kohtuus (2006) *STAKES asiantuntijaraportti*, Helsinki: STAKES.

Oliver, A., Mossialos, E. and Wilsford, D. (2005) 'Special issue: legacies and latitude in European health policy', *Journal of Health Politics, Policy and Law*, 30(1–2).

Ollila, E. and Koivusalo, M. (2002) 'The World Health Report 2000: the World Health Organization health policy steering off course – changed values, poor evidence, and lack of accountability', *International Journal of Health Services*, 32(3): 503–514.

Opinion Leader Research (2006) *Your Health, Your Care, Your Say: Research Report for the Department of Health*, London: Opinion Leader Research.

Organization for Economic Cooperation and Development (OECD) (1992) *The Reform of Health Care: A Comparative Analysis of Seven OECD Countries*, Paris: OECD.

—— (1994) *The Reform of Health Care Systems: A Review of Seventeen OECD Countries*, Paris: OECD.

—— (1995) *New Directions in Health Policy*, Paris: OECD.

—— (1996) *The Will to Change*, Paris: OECD.

—— (1997) *OECD Report on Regulatory Reform*, Synthesis Report, Paris: OECD, http://www.oecd.org/datadecd/17/25/2391768.pdf (accessed 12 April 2009).

—— (1998) *Multilateral Agreement on Investment, Draft consolidated text*, DAFFE/MAI(98)7/REV1, Paris: OECD.

—— (2003a) *Health Care Systems: Lessons From the Reform Experience*, Paris: OECD.

—— (2005) *Finland*, Paris: OECD.

—— (2007) *Achieving Results for Sustained Growth: OECD Country Reviews of Regulatory Reform*, Paris: OECD.

—— (2008) *Pharmaceutical Pricing Policies in a Global Market*, OECD Health Policy Studies, 24 September 2008, Paris: OECD.

Orme, J. (2001) 'Regulation or fragmentation? Directions for social work under new labour', *British Journal of Social Work*, 31(4): 611–624.

Orme, J., Powell, J., Taylor, P., Harrison, T. and Grey, M. (eds) (2003) *Public Health for the 21ˢᵗ Century: New Perspectives on Policy, Participation and Practice*, Maidenhead: Open University Press.

Ortino, F. (2006) 'Treaty interpretation and the WTO appellate body report in the US-Gambling: A critique', *Journal of International Economic Law*, 9(1): 117–148.

Osborne, D. and Gaebler, T. (1992) *Reinventing Government*, New York: Addison-Wesley.

Oxley, H. and MacFarlan, M. (1995) 'Healthcare reform: controlling spending and increasing efficiency', *OECD Economic Studies* 24, Paris: OECD.

Palola, E. (2007) *FC sisämarkkinat*, Helsinki: Sosiaali- ja terveysturvan keskusliitto.

Partanen, M-L. and Martikainen, T. (1994) 'Finns defined patients' rights before Dutch', *British Medical Journal*, 309(6947): 130–131.

Paton, C. (2000) 'New Labour, new health policy?', in A. Hann (ed.) *Analysing Health Policy*, Aldershot: Ashgate Publishing.

Pauwelyn, J. (2005) 'Rien ne va plus? Distinguishing domestic regulation from market access in GATT and GATS', *World Trade Review*, 4(2): 131–170.

Peckham, S. (2004) 'Health tourism: a threat to international health equity', *Health Matters*, 37, December.

Pekurinen, M., Punkar, i M. and Pokka, M. (1997) *Asiakkaiden valinnanvapauden toteutuminen Suomen terveydenhuollossa*, Helsinki: Sosiaali- ja terveysministeriön monisteita 1997: 16.

Pierre, J. (1993) 'Legitimacy, institutional change, and the politics of public administration', *International Political Science* Review, 14(4): 387–401.

Pollit, C. and Bouckaert, C. (2004) *Public Management Reforms: A Comparative Analysis*, Oxford: Oxford University Press.

Pollock, A. M. (2004) *NHS Plc: The Privatisation of Our Healthcare*, London: Verso.

Pollock, A.M. and Price, D. (2000) 'Trading public health for private wealth', *The Lancet* 356(9246): 1941.

Praktikertjänst (2008) We are praktikertjänst, http://www.praktikertjanst.se/templates/Page.aspx?id=14 (accessed 16 December 2008).

Pratchett, L. (2004) 'Local autonomy, local democracy and the "new localism"', *Political Studies*, 52(2): 358–375.

Premfors, R. (1998) 'Reshaping the democratic state: Swedish experiences in a comparative perspective', *Public Administration*, 6(1):141–159.

Prior, L. (2003) 'Belief, knowledge and expertise: the emergence of the lay expert in medical sociology', *Sociology of Health and Illness*, 25 (Silver Anniversary Issue): 41–57.

Piore, M. and Sabel, C. (1986) *The Second Industrial Divide: Possibilities for Prosperity*, New York: Basic Books.

Propper, C., Wilson, D. and Burgess, S. (2005) 'Extending choice in English healthcare: the implications of the economic evidence', *CMPO Working Paper Series 05/133*, Bristol: Centre for Market and Public Organisation.

Protocol on the exercise of shared competence (2007) 'Protocol on the exercise of shared competence', *Official Journal of the European Union* C306/158, Brussels: European Union.

Reform (2008) 'Doctors for Reform response to the top-up review', Reform Bulletin 4 November, London: Reform, http://www.reform.co.uk/doctorsforreformresponsetothetopupreview_501.php (accessed 12 April 2009).

Regeringens Proposition (1997) *Patientens ställning*, 1997/98: 189.

—— (1998) *Stärkt patientinflytande*, 1998/99: 4

—— (2004) *Driftsformer för offentligt finansierade sjukhus*, 2004/05: 105.

—— (2007) *Driftsformer för sjukhus*, 2006/07: 52.

—— (2008a) *Lag om valfrihetssystem*, 2008/09: 29.

—— (2008b) *Vårdval I primärvården*, 2008/09: 74.

Richards, M. (2008) Letter on Consequences of Additional Private Drugs for NHS Care, RichardsM1-week (Gateway Number 10171), London: Department of Health.

Richards, T. (1999) 'New EU health commissioner airs his priorities', *British Medical Journal*, 319(7211): 662.

Rodrik, D. (2007) 'Saving globalisation from its cheerleaders', July 2008, http://ksghome.harvard.edu/~drodrik/Saving%20globalization.pdf (accessed 15 December 2008).

Romanow, R. J. (2002) *Building on Values: The Future of Health Care in Canada Final Report*, Ottawa: Commission on the Future of Health Care in Canada.

Romppainen, E. (2003) *Raha-automaattiyhdistys ja kilpailu*, Helsinki: RAY.

Rosen, P. (2006) 'Public dialogue on healthcare prioritisation', *Health Policy*, 79(1): 107–116.

Rosenmöller, M., McKee, M. and Baeten, R. (eds) (2006) *Patient Mobility in the European Union: Learning from Experience*, Copenhagen: World Health Organisation on behalf of Europe 4 Patients project and the European Observatory on Health Systems and Policies.

Rosenthal, M. (1986) 'Beyond equity: Swedish health policy and the private sector', *The Millbank Quarterly*, 64(4): 592–621.

Rouvinen, P., Saranummi, N., Lammi M (eds) (1995) *Terveydenhuolto versoo teollisuutta – hyvinvointiklusterin kilpailukyky*, Helsinki: ETLA.

Saarinen, A. (2007a) 'Markkinat ja lääkäriprofessio, Suomen Lääkäriliiton ideat suhteessa markkinoistumiseen julkisessa terveydenhuoltojärjestelmässä vuosina 1970–2005', *Yhteiskuntapolitiikka*, 72(6): 121–136.

—— (2007b) 'Lääkärien mielipiteet terveydenhuollon markkinoistumisesta', *Yhteiskuntapolitiikka*, 72(6): 599–612.

Saint-Martin, D. (1998) 'The New Managerialism and the policy influence of consultants in government: an historical-institutionalist analysis of Britain, Canada and France', *Governance*, 11(3) 319–356.

Saltman, R. B. (1994) 'Patient choice and patient empowerment in Northern European health systems: A conceptual framework', *International Journal of Health Services*, 24(2): 201–229.

—— (2002) 'Regulating the incentives: the past and present role of the state in healthcare systems', *Social Science and Medicine*, 54(1): 1677–1684.

Saltman, R. B. and Otter, C. v. (1987) 'Re-vitalising public healthcare systems: a proposal for public competition in Sweden', *Health Policy*, 7(1): 21–40.

—— (1989) 'Voice, choice and the question of CMI democracy in the Swedish welfare state', *Economic and Industrial Democracy*, 10(2): 195–209.

—— (1992) *Planned Markets and Public Competition: Strategic Reform in Northern European Health Systems*, Buckingham: Open University Press.

Saltman, R. B. and Figueras, J. (eds) (1997) *European Health Care Reform: Analysis of Current Strategies*, Copenhagen: World Health Organization Regional Office for Europe.

Saltman, R. B., Figueras, J. and Sakellarides, C. (1998) *Health Care Reform in Europe*, Basingstoke: Open University Press.

Saravia, N. G. and Miranda, J. F. (2004) 'Plumbing the brain drain', *Bulletin of the World Health Organisation*, 82(8): 608–613.

Scholte, J. A. (2001) *Globalisation: A Critical Introduction*, Basingstoke: Palgrave.

Shaw, J. and Baker, M. (2004) '"Expert Patient" – dream or nightmare?', *British Medical Journal*, 328(7442): 723–724.

Sheldon, T. (1994) 'Dutch law defines patients' rights', *British Medical Journal*, 308: 616.

Sirnö, M. (2006) *Lakialoite*, Laki potilaan asemasta ja oikeuksista annetun lain muuttamisesta, LA 20/2006.

Sjukvårdspartiet (2008) Ett rikspolitisk handlingsprogramm för ett nationellt sjukvårdsparti, http://www.sjukvardspartiet.org/SVPr/Om_oss.html   Printed 12.12. 2008 (accessed 15 December 2008).

SKL (2004) *Orimliga konsekvenser av EU:s arbetsmarknadsdirektiv. Pressmeddelande*, Stockholm: Svenska kommunförbyndet och Lansdsingsförbundget.

Slote Morris, Z. and Dawson, S. (2006) *Policy Futures for UK Health: Discussion Paper and Review of Current and Proposed Public Health Policy*, Nuffield Institute, Judge Business School, Cambridge: University of Cambridge.

Smith, K. and Sheaff, R. (2000) 'Some are more equal than others: differing levels of representation in primary care groups', in A. Hann (ed.) (2000) *Analysing Health Policy*, Aldershot: Ashgate Publishing.

Smith v. North East Derbyshire Primary Care Trust (2006) EWCA civ 1291 [23 August 2006].

Socialdepartement (2007) *Komittedirektiv- patientents rätt till vården*, Dir 2007: 90.

Socialstyrelsen (1992) *Husläkare – för kontinuitet och trygghet i vården*, Stockholm: Socialstyrelsen.

Somerset Health and Social Care NHS Trust (2008) http://www.somerset.nhs.uk/ news_info/involvement/index.html (accessed 5 July 2008).

SOU (1993) *Hälso och sjukvården i framtiden: tre modeller: Rapport från expert-gruppen*. Stockholm: SOU.

—— (1994) *Sjukvårdsreformer i andra länder*, SOU: 15.

—— (1995) *Vårdens svåra val*, SOU: 5.

—— (1996) *Behov och resurser i vården. En analys*, SOU: 163.

—— (1997) *Patienten har rätt*, SOU: 154.

—— (1999a) *God vård på lika villkor. Om statens styrning av hälso-och sjukvården*, SOU: 66.

—— (1999b) *Upphandling av hälsö och sjukvårdstjänster*, SOU: 149.

—— (2002) *Vinst för värden*, SOU 2002: 31.

—— (2008a) *Lov att välja*, SOU 2008: 16.

—— (2008b) *Vårdval i Sverige*, SOU 2008: 37.

Stahl, T., Wismar, M., Ollila, E., Lahtinen, E. and Leppo, K. (2006) *Health in all Policies: Prospects and Potentials* (EU Public Health Programme), Helsinki: Finnish Ministry of Social Affairs and Health.

STAKES (2007) *Statistical Yearbook on Social Welfare and Health Care 2007*, Helsinki: National Research and Development Centre for Welfare and Health.

—— (2008) *Statistical Yearbook on Social Welfare and Health Care 2008*, Helsinki: National Research and Development Centre for Welfare and Health.

Stewart, M. (2001) 'Towards a global definition of patient centred care', *British Medical Journal*, 322(7284): 444–445.

Stewart, J. (2003) *Modernising British Local Government: An Assessment of Labour's Reform Programme*, Basingstoke: Palgrave.

Stillwell, B., Diallo, K., Zurn, P., Vujicic, M., Adams, O. and Dal Poz, M. (2004) 'Migration of health-care workers from developing countries: strategic approaches to its management', *Bulletin of World Health Organisation*, 82(8): 595–600.

STM (1998) Ministry of Social Affairs and Health, Terveydenhuollon kehittämispro-jekti, Selvitysmiesraportti 1, *Asiakkaan asema terveydenhuollossa*, Työryhmämuistioita 1998: 1.

—— (2001) *Report on the Use of State Subsidy for Child and Adolescent Psychiatry in the Year 2000*, Helsinki: Ministry of Social Affairs and Health.

—— (2002) *Decision in Principle by the Council of State on Securing the Future of Health Care*, Helsinki: Ministry of Social Affairs and Health.

—— (2004) *Health Care in Finland*, Brochures of the Ministry of Social Affairs and Health, 2004: 11.

—— (2008a) *Final Report to the Monitoring Group on the National Health Care Project Actions in 2002–2007*, Helsinki: Ministry of Social Affairs and Health.

—— (2008b) Ministry of Social Affairs and Health, *Proposal for expanding vouchers, Palvelusetelin käyttöalan laajentaminen*. Palvelusetelityöryhmän muistio. Sosiaali-ja terveysministeriön selvityksiä 2008: 32.

—— (2008c) Ministry of Social Affairs and Health, *Proposal for Health Services Law*, Helsinki: Ministry of Social Affairs and Health.

Stocking, B. (1991) 'Patient's Charter', *British Medical Journal*, 303(6811): 1148–1149.

Strong, P. and Robinson, J. (1990) *The NHS Under New Management*, Buckingham: Open University Press.

Swedish Institute (2003) 'Healthcare in Sweden', cited in M. Fotaki (2007), pp. 1059–1075.

TEHY (2008) *Kuntavaaliteemat 2008*, Paras äänestää nyt hyvän hoidon puolesta, www.tehy.fi/tehy_vaikuttajana/tutkimukset_ja_selvitykset/vuosi_2008 (accessed 15 December 2008).

TEKES (2008) *New Methods in Developing Social and Health Care Services*, Helsinki: TEKES.

Terveystalo (2008*)* 'Largest shareholders', http://www.terveystalo.com/WebRoot/100979/Yksileveys.aspx?id=1019988 (accessed 12 December 2008).

Thorlby, R. (2006) *Where the Patient was King? A Study of Patient Choice and its Effect on Five Specialist HIV Units in London*, London: King's Fund.

TIMBRO (2005) 'Vårdkonton. Ett enkelt steg mot billigare sjukvård', *Timbro Briefing Paper 4*, Stockholm: TIMBRO.

Timonen, V. (2003) *Restructuring the Welfare State: Globalization and Social Policy Reform in Finland and Sweden*, Cheltenham: Edward Elgar.

Topf, R. (1995) 'Electoral participation', in H.-D. Klingemann and D. Fuchs (eds) *Citizens and the State*, Oxford: Oxford University Press.

Trafford Healthcare NHS Trust (2006) Public consultation on the provision of Inpatient Beds at Altrincham General Hospital, (http://www.trafford.nhs.uk/TraffordWebPortal/cmsitem?documentPath=Public%20consultation%20on%20the%20provision%20of%20Inpatient%20Beds%20at%20Altrincham%20G (accessed 13 December 2008).

Treaty of Nice (2001) Consolidated version of the Treaty Establishing the European Community, *Official Journal* C 325, 24 December 2002.

Treaty of Lisbon (2007) Consolidated versions of the Treaty on European Union and the Treaty on the Functioning of European Union, Council of the European Union, 66/55/08 rev 1, Brussels 30 April 2008.

Tritter, J. (1994) 'The citizen's charter: opportunities for users' perspectives', *The Political Quarterly*, 654(4): 397–414.

—— (2008) '"Getting to know myself": changing needs and gaining knowledge among people with cancer', in E. Denny and S. Earle (eds) *Long Term Conditions and Nursing Practice*, Basingstoke: Palgrave.

Tritter, J. and McCallum, A. (2006) 'The snakes and ladders of user involvement: moving beyond Arnstein', *Health Policy*, 76(2): 156–168.

Tritter, J., Daykin, N., Evans, S. and Sanidas, M. (2003) *Improving Cancer Services Through Patient Involvement*, Oxford: Radcliffe Medical Press.

Twaddle, A.C. (1999) *Health Care Reform in Sweden 1980–1994*, London: Auburn House.

UNCTAD/WHO (1998) *International Trade in Health Service: A Development Perspective*, Geneva: UNCTAD/WHO.

United Nations Economic Commission for Europe (1998) *Convention on Access to Information, Public Participation in Decision-Making and Access to Justice in Environmental Matters,* Aarhus: UNECE.

UNHCHR (1966) *International Covenant on Economic, Social and Cultural Rights,* http://www.unhchr.ch/html/menu3/b/a_cescr.htm (accessed 14 April 2008).

United States Department of the Treasury (2008) HSAs Frequently Asked Questions, http://www.ustreas.gov/offices/public-affairs/hsa/faq_basics.shtml (accessed 23 July 2008). See also http://www.hsainsider.com.

Uusitalo, H. (1996) 'Economic crisis and social policy in Finland in the 1990s', *Social Policy Research Centre*, Discussion Paper No. 70, Sydney: SPRC.

Valentine, N., Darby, C. and Bonsel, G.J. (2008) 'Which aspects of non-clinical quality of care are most important? Results from WHO's general population surveys of "health systems responsiveness" in 41 countries', *Social Science and Medicine*, 66(9): 1939–1950.

Vallgårda, S., Krasnick, A. and Vrangbæk, K. (2001) *Denmark: Healthcare Systems in Transition*, Copenhagen: European Observatory on Healthcare Systems.

Valtioneuvosto (2004) *Osaava, avautuva ja uudistuva Suomi. Suomi maailmantaloudessa – selvityksen loppuraportti*, Valtioneuvoston kanslian julkaisusarja 19/2994, Helsinki: Valtioneuvoston kanslia.

—— (2006) Talousneuvoston sihteeristön globalisaatioselvitys: Suomen vastaus globalisaation haasteeseen, Valioneuvoston kanslian julkaisusarja 17/2006.

Valtioneuvoston asetus (2004) Hoitoonpääsyn toteuttamisesta ja alueellisesta yhteistyöstä, 1019/24, Helsinki: Ministry of Social Affairs and Health.

Valvira (2009a) 'Effectiveness through supervision', http://www.valvira.fi/en/about_valvira (accessed 14 April 2009).

—— (2009b) 'Terveydenhuollon valvonta', http://www.valvira.fi/files/Liite3_Terveydenhuollon_valvonta.pdf (accessed 14 April 2009).

Vanhanen, M. (2004) *Vanhanen government programme*, Helsinki: Valtioneuvosto.

Viidas, K. and Nilsson, J. (2007) 'Öka konsumenttnyttan I vård och omsorg – förslag till konkurrens och ökat företagande', *Konkurrensverkets Rapportserie 3*, Stockholm: konkurrensverket.

Vos, P. (2002) *Health and Healthcare in the Netherlands*, Maarssen: Elsevier gezonheidszorg.

Vuorenkoski, L. (2008) *Health Care Systems in Transition: Finland*, Brussels: European Observatory on Health Care Systems.

Vågerö, D. (1994) 'Equity and efficiency in health reform: a European view', *Social Science and Medicine*, 39(9): 1203–1210.

Waitzkin, H. (1994) 'The strange career of managed competition: from military failure to medical success?', *American Journal of Public Health*, 84(3): 482–489.

Walker, D. (2005) 'New new localism: a seismic shift in local government?', The *Guardian*, 2 March, http://www.guardian.co.uk/society/Mar/02/politics.localgovernment (accessed 15 April 2009).

Whitehead M, Gustaffson R, Diderichsen F (1997) 'Why is Sweden rethinking its NH-style reforms?', *British Medical Journal,* 315: 935–939.

Williams, M. (1998) *Voice, Trust and Memory: Marginalised Groups and the Failure of Liberal Representation*, Princeton, NJ: Princeton University Press.

Winblad, U. (2007) 'Valfirheten: en misslychad sjukvårdsreform?', in P. Blomqvist (ed.) *Vem Styr Vården? Organisation och Politisk Styrning Inom Svensk Sjukvård*, Stockholm: SNS Förlag.

Winblad-Spånberg, U. (2003) *Från beslut till verklighet. Läkarnas roll vid implementering av valfrihetsreformer I hälso- och sjukvården*, Uppsala Universitet, Stockholm: Elanders Gotab.

World Health Organisation (WHO) (1948) *Constitution of the WHO*, Geneva: WHO.

—— (1986) *The Ottawa Charter for Health Promotion*, First International Conference on Health Promotion, Ottawa, Canada 21 November, http://www.who.int/hpr/NPH/ docs/ottawa_charter_hp.pdf (accessed 14 April 2009).

—— (1991) *Sundsvall Statement on Supportive Environments for Health: Third International Conference on Health Promotion*, Sundsvall, Sweden.

—— (2000) *World Health Report. Health Systems: Improving Performance*, Geneva: WHO.

—— (2002) '25 Questions and answers on health and human rights', *Health & Human Rights Publication Series*, Issue 1, July, Geneva: WHO.

—— (2006) *World Health Report*, Geneva: WHO.

—— (2008a) *World Health Report*, Geneva: WHO.

—— (2008b) *Closing the Gap in a Generation: Health Equity Through Action on the Social Determinants of Health, Final Report of the Commission on Social Determinants of Health*, Geneva: WHO.

World Health Organisation Regional Office for Europe (1985) *Targets for Health for All: Targets in Support of the European Regional Strategy for Health for All*, Copenhagen: WHO Regional Office for Europe.

—— (1994) *Declaration on the Promotion of Patients' Rights in Europe*, Copenhagen: WHO Regional Office for Europe.

—— (1996) 'The Ljubljana Charter on reforming healthcare', *British Medical Journal*, 312: 1664–1665.

WHO/UNICEF (1978a) *Alma-Ata 1978: Primary Health Care: Report of the International Conference on Primary Health Care*, Alma-Ata, USSR, 6–12 September 1978, Geneva: WHO.

—— (1978b) *Declaration of Alma-Ata*, Geneva: WHO.

World Medical Association (WMA) (2005) 'World Medical Association Declaration on the Rights of the Patient', http://www.wma.net/e/policy/l4.htm (accessed 19 July 2008).

World Trade Organisation (2001) *Declaration on the TRIPS agreement and public health* (WT/MIN(01)/DEC/W/2), Ministerial Conference, Doha, 9–14 November.

—— (2005) *United States: Measures Affecting the Cross-Border Supply of Gambling and Betting Services, WT/DS285/AB/R*, Washington: World Trade Organisation.

—— (2008) 'Disciplines on domestic regulation pursuant to GATS Article IV: 4', World Trade Organisation Working Party on domestic regulation, Room document, Revised Draft informal note by the chairman, 23 January, Geneva: WTO.

—— (2009) 'Services commitments on the basis of WTO services database', http://tsdb.wto.org/default.aspx (accessed 14 April 2009).

Zalmanov, Y. (1997) 'Some antecedents to healthcare reform: Israel and the United States', *Policy and Politics*, 25(3): 251–268.

Index

Milton Keynes UK
Ingram Content Group UK Ltd.
UKHW040058071024
449327UK00019B/632

9 780415 612050